The CSA Exam

Maximizing your success

The CSA Exam

Maximizing your success

Rachel Roberts
David Russell
Simon Ormerod
Anjum Iqbal

WILEY Blackwell

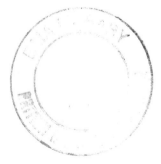

Registered office: John Wiley & Sons, Ltd, The Atrium, Southern Gate, Chichester, West Sussex, PO19 8SQ, UK
Editorial offices: 9600 Garsington Road, Oxford, OX4 2DQ, UK
The Atrium, Southern Gate, Chichester, West Sussex, PO19 8SQ, UK
1606 Golden Aspen Drive, Suites 103 and 104, Ames, Iowa 50010, USA

For details of our global editorial offices, for customer services and for information about how to apply for permission to reuse the copyright material in this book please see our website at www.wiley.com/wiley-blackwell

Library of Congress Cataloging-in-Publication Data applied for.

ISBN: 9781119079194

A catalogue record for this book is available from the British Library.

Wiley also publishes its books in a variety of electronic formats. Some content that appears in print may not be available in electronic books.

Cover image: © KrulUA/Gettyimages

Set in 9.5/12pt MinionPro by SPi Global, Chennai, India
Printed and bound in Malaysia by Vivar Printing Sdn Bhd

1 2016

Contents

PART TWO A 'PALETTE' OF 16 CSA-TYPE CASES AND 6 ETHICAL CASES

About the companion website

The companion website contains a number of resources, including 18 clips – 12 cases + 6 ethical dilemmas, general suggestions on making the best use of the clips and the video- and case-specific educational support material.

www.wiley.com\go\Roberts\CSAExam

About the authors

Rachel Roberts

Rachel is a GP, trainer, CSA examiner, and is a Patch Associate Director for General Practice, London. She is also the Associate Director for trainees in difficulty for North East and Central London. Her main interests are in helping learners to achieve their full potential and to enjoy working in a typical, busy general practice.

David Russell

As a retired teacher, David has a strong educational and examining background. Appointed Lay Adviser to the RCGP, he worked on the Simulated Surgery Exams and, subsequently, on the development of the CSA exam. He has been the CSA Role-Player Lead, responsible for the training and quality assurance of the simulated patients, and has published several papers about his work with the simulated 'patients' in the CSA.

Simon Ormerod

Simon is a GP with a special interest in General Practice. He has been a trainer since 1996, and a member of the MRCGP examiners panel since 2010. He is currently Honorary Secretary of the North East London Faculty RCGP.

Anjum Iqbal

Anjum qualified from the Royal Free Hospital and worked as a GP for 5 years in Stepney, East London. In 1996, he moved GP practice to Enfield, North London. He remains committed to Education and Training as a Trainer and Programme Director in Enfield. He has also been a CSA examiner since 2008. It remains a privilege for him to serve patients and enjoy consulting.

Acknowledgements

The authors would like to acknowledge the North East London faculty of the RCGP, and Anwar Khan, who brought the team together in organizing the RCGP course. Working together on this course, being GP educators and being examiners for the RCGP were the breeding ground for the ideas in this book.

We would also like to thank those who contributed to early versions of course material from all London faculties and the RCGP. They are Anwar Khan, Mei-Ling Denney and Marilyn Graham. We would like to thank Dr Anwar Khan for the ideas that developed into the six ethical case clips.

Foreword

The Clinical Skills Assessment (CSA) is less than a decade old. But during that time, it has continued to evolve to keep abreast of the latest in best practice in assessment. It has also been at the centre of a storm of controversy relating to differential pass rates for those who trained abroad and UK graduates from BME backgrounds. While the recent judicial review found no evidence of discrimination, it remains the case that the CSA is a challenge for many aspiring to be General Practitioners in the United Kingdom.

For those looking for a magic formula through the CSA, take note, you will be disappointed. Equally, this book does not offer a recipe for passing the examination. However, if you want to understand the essence of being a sophisticated consulter in a modern-day general practice, this book opens a world of opportunities. This book offers you three opportunities – the first is for you to learn about yourselves (what are your needs, how might you learn, where can you look to learn about the CSA and who can support you in your learning journey); the second is to make the most of the learning opportunities that general practice training has to offer; and the final is to demystify the CSA itself.

The chapters are written in an easy-to-read manner with a strong emphasis on simplifying the language around the CSA, a focus on bringing out the practical tips to maximize your learning and opportunities for improving your consulting. It reconnects the CSA with the best in educational practice, and in doing so, re-frames the CSA – not as an examination to be feared but to be seen as the culmination of a year-long (and career-long) expression of mingling the science of modern medical practice with compassionate consulting.

Three of the authors of this book are practising GPs – they apply the art of compassionate consulting and modern medicine in their day-to-day practice. They are all educators – they understand the challenges of preparing doctors for a life of general practice (not just preparing for the examination but for a career of consulting). The doctors are all CSA examiners – they know how examiners think and what they expect. In addition, Dave Russell has been the role-player lead for the CSA, who has a wealth of understanding around the simulated patient.

This book is the accumulation of their collective experience, their desire to show you that there is an alternative to learning focused on 'getting through the exam', and by doing so they are trying to achieve something greater – make effective consulting part of your daily practice and, by doing so, reduce the tension and anxiety associated with the CSA.

But don't just believe what I say! Dip into the book, read a couple of chapters and even try out some of the suggestions the authors make. It has the potential to transform how you do things in the consulting room!

Dr Sanjiv Ahluwalia MBBS FRCGP MSc
Head of Primary Care Education and Development
Health Education North Central and East London

Part One

Introduction

How to use this book to maximize success in your CSA exam

In planning this book, we aim to help you understand more about the three main components of the CSA exam, and to give insights into how you can maximize your potential for success.

Firstly, we will consider your own personal needs, as the *C*andidate, in order to pass the exam. Secondly, we will discuss getting the most from your *S*imulated patients (the role-players). Then we will give you an overview of the *A*ssessment itself – what to expect and what is expected of you.

Each of these first three chapters contains boxes of essential 'Learning Points', and after each one we have listed as bullet points relevant 'Tips and Hints' under the headings of 'Getting Started', 'The Consultation' and 'On the Day'. We hope you will find all these useful in your studies as a guide and aide-memoire.

Example:

CSA Preparation with This Book

- Part 1 will help you to develop as a Candidate, understand the *S*imulated patients and how the *A*ssessors mark.
- Part 2 gives cases with detailed mark schedules, ideally to role play in pairs and groups.
- Part 3 is an interactive website, including role played introductions to cases, for you to watch, and continue the role play. Material to help you assess and analyse the consultations is included.

The CSA Exam: Maximizing your Success, First Edition. Rachel Roberts.

Companion Website: www.wiley.com\go\Roberts\CSAExam

We go on to give advice about dealing with dilemmas and applying an ethical approach in your consultations. We suggest an exercise to put all this into practice, and then go on to supplement this with a focus on CSA examiner feedback. Chapter 7 reviews possible areas of concern and how to avoid and/or deal with them. Part 1 concludes with a collation of the essential Learning Points from the earlier chapters.

In Part 2, we have collaborated to produce 16 cases to help you practise your exam technique, and perhaps to use as a template to apply to the exercise suggested in Chapter 5 creating your own cases, focusing on identified hot topics. In addition we have 6 ethical cases with supporting material in chapter 4.

Finally, in addition to the written materials in this book, we have filmed 18 clips – 12 cases + 6 ethical dilemmas to offer an additional learning resource. This gives a different perspective on the six cases illustrating ethical dilemmas in Chapter 4 of Part 1 and on 12 of the cases in Part 2. Purchasers of the book will have the opportunity to access these video clips on our website, and details of how we recommend they could be used are outlined in the Introduction to Part 2.

We hope you find this approach useful, and that our advice helps you to maximize your potential in the CSA. The RCGP demographic is changing since the MRCGP has become mandatory and the functions of the College are changing too. At its core remains the function of ensuring high-quality, professional GP care for all patients, and the MRCGP exam is essential to this. Patients need value-driven, patient-centred, quality- and safety-focused, energetic, knowledgeable, vocational doctors LIKE YOU!

Good luck!

Rachel Roberts
David Russell
Simon Ormerod
Anjum Iqbal

Chapter 1 **Maximizing your potential in the CSA**

In planning this book, we aim to help you understand more about three main areas. Firstly, your own personal needs in order to pass the exam. Secondly, how to get the most from your 'patients' or role-players, and thirdly, how to understand more about the exam itself. This chapter addresses how you can develop to your full potential in the CSA exam and beyond. We cover how to assess your own needs in terms of knowledge, consultation skills and also, very importantly, the preparation needed for maximizing your performance on the day. The goal of passing the CSA may be the initial motivator to develop these areas. Our real hope, however, is that you come to see your journey to success in the CSA as an excellent preparation for your life as a GP. We expect you to go on, equipped with your skills, to be successful in General Practice.

The aim of this chapter is to suggest resources for you to assess your needs, identify any potential barriers to passing the CSA and generate strategies to overcome any such barriers. This will result in drawing up a 'CSA PDP' to use and put into practice in the weeks or months before the exam. Practice of both consulting strategies and psychological strategies for dealing with stress, so as to focus purely on the 'patient', will, therefore, be honed and your all-round potential maximized in time for the exam.

Take this moment to note down any areas where you feel less confident, and so to begin to draft your CSA PDP

Thoughts such as
'I hope undiagnosed vaginal bleeding, or Parkinson's disease, doesn't come up',
are a good place to start making your planning list.

The CSA Exam: Maximizing your Success, First Edition. Rachel Roberts.

Companion Website: www.wiley.com\go\Roberts\CSAExam

Think of your last difficult consultation, for example an angry or very anxious patient, and add that to your development list.
Think of the last patient who left your room less than satisfied, and add the possible reasons to your wish list to practise.

When doing an assessment of your educational needs, it is important to focus equally on the clinical aspects of general practice as well as on interpersonal skills. This is reflected in both the marking schedules and the college motto *Cum Scientia Caritas*, 'science with compassion'. The assistance of your trainer/educational supervisor in assessing your educational needs is paramount, as they will often have had the benefit of working with many other learners in order to form an opinion. Your Programme Directors may be valuable resources too, as, of course, are your peers on your VTS, in helping you build on your strengths and identify areas for improvement in terms of knowledge and competence.

Knowledge

Assessing your knowledge base is something you may have done at the start of your registrar year by self-rating, and also after a discussion with your trainer. This activity should lead to an educational plan. A month or 2 before the CSA is an ideal time to revisit this process, taking into account the current GP curriculum and any 'Hot Topics'. A number of tools exist – for example the RCGP 'Condensed Curriculum Guide self assessment scale'. This is available online, via the RCGP website, and can be purchased from the RCGP Bookshop.

It covers knowledge, skills and attitudes. A number of other possible rating scales exist – anything which accurately covers the curriculum will be fine, if the layout suits you. Patients themselves are an excellent resource. By identifying *patient unmet needs (PUNs)* in your consultations, you will identify your *doctor's educational needs (DENs)* – (Eve, 2003).

Time now to do a brief knowledge-base assessment to confirm areas of the curriculum needing attention

Ideally 1–2 months before the CSA exam:

- Use one of the GP curriculum confidence rating scales.
- Write the areas needing development in your CSA PDP form, at the end of this chapter.

Having decided any areas for development, these can be entered in your 'CSA PDP'. Following this, a strategy for improving these areas and potential resources for doing so can be listed.

LEARNING POINT 1: 'My CSA PDP' – resources for improvement

- RCGP e-modules EKU (Essential Knowledge Updates) are compiled by representatives of the examiners' panel.
- 'Innovait' – covers every section of the Curriculum on a 3 yearly cycle (ST1-3).
- Summaries of GP guidelines such as 'e-guidelines' which also produce a book with a compilation of current guidance in handy flow charts and tables.
- GP free magazines which include CPD or review articles, for example 'Prescriber' magazine.
- 'PUNs and DENs' after each surgery, with a quick reference to the current guidelines after seeing patients.

A tip we often give is to repeat an AKT test or two in the month or so before the exam – this may expose gaps in your learning and is likely to prompt you to polish areas that may be hotter topics.

Consultation skills

From the analysis of the feedback to candidates given by examiners during the marking process, we know which areas of the consultation are highlighted most commonly, and are, thus, the areas most likely to cause you difficulty in the CSA.

The first aim of this section, therefore, is to help you identify potential barriers to passing the CSA, and hence make plans to maximize your potential. Secondly, we will summarise the most successful ways you can develop awareness of your consultation style. Finally, but possibly most importantly, this section will raise awareness of behavioural theories, which help interpersonal interaction, and, therefore, have the potential to improve your patient consultations. Such skills can most certainly be learnt, but only with practice and feedback from your patients and educators.

LEARNING POINT 2: Examiners' feedback statements – areas commonly highlighted by examiners as needing improvement

- Consultation structure/time management.
- Management plans in keeping with current best practice.

- Identifying the patient's agenda, health beliefs and preferences.
- Use of verbal and non-verbal cues. Active listening.
- Sharing the management plan, clarifying the roles of doctor and patient (RCGP, 2014; Trafford, 2010).

Issues with structure can be addressed by watching your own videos, and analysing the sections of the consultation, using any of your favoured consultation models. Comparing your consultations against consultation models and also against the feedback statements may highlight for you which areas of the consultation are receiving least attention, and, therefore, need developing. Commonly, during the time-limited CSA consultations, candidates spend too long on data-gathering, leaving little time for the management plan, and even less for sharing ideas with the patient around the management plan. This is emphasised in the recent consultation model, 'The Consultation Hill' by McKelvey (2010), which refers to the preparation for the CSA in terms of managing 10-minute consultations and leaving sufficient time for these vital sections.

The feedback statement given to a candidate – '*Does not develop a management plan (including prescribing and referral) that is appropriate and in line with current best practice*' – suggests that the knowledge base needs addressing. In a sense, it should be possible for all candidates to remedy this, using the methods mentioned in the 'Knowledge' section. Practice in applying the knowledge is required, as real patients are generally far more complicated than the guidelines suggest, often having multi-morbidity or important influencing factors in their social situations. Hence, discussion of cases with your trainer and practice/community team colleagues, and also checking that knowledge is truly sound, will improve these areas. Examples could include being aware of prescribing for the presenting condition safely, but in order to do this, you may have to take into account a patient's other medical conditions, or occupation, which would influence appropriate or safe choices (e.g. prescribing in safety critical jobs such as tube train drivers, or in pregnancy).

The feedback statements – '*Does not identify the patient's agenda, health beliefs and preferences*', and also '*poor active listening and use of cues*' – are at the heart of interpersonal skills during the data-gathering section of the consultation in particular. Here, GP consultation models as well as other simple behavioural models can be extremely effective in GP consultations, particularly with role-played CSA cases. Such behavioural or neurolinguistic models give us some very useful pointers to consulting effectively –

- Become interested and curious
- Create rapport
- Ask questions
- *Listen* and check your understanding of what they describe
- Pay particular attention to their non-verbal communication
- *Leave enough time for management* (adapted from Reg Connolly + Pegasus NLP, 2014 for the GP consultation by Dr R Roberts)

For example, if you ask a person presenting with headaches how things are at home, and there is an immediate break in eye contact, and a change in posture to become more closed, it would suggest that home may be an area of pain or discomfort for the patient.

LEARNING POINT 3: Tips for effective consulting style in the CSA

- Become interested and curious.
- Create rapport.
- Ask questions.
- *Listen* and check your understanding of what the patient describes.
- Pay particular attention to the patient's non-verbal communication.

'*Does not develop a SHARED management plan, or clarify the roles of doctor and patient*' applies the above principles to the discussion with the patient regarding the suggested management plan. For example, "be curious" about what they think of the plan or the options you have given them. You are then in a position to adapt and negotiate. Again, work in behavioural techniques suggests the following:

- 'In any interaction, the person with the greatest behavioural flexibility has the most influence on outcome'.
- 'Discover the person's perceptions before you seek to influence them' (Connolly/Pegasus, 2014).

Our interpretation of this, in relation to our consultations, and particularly the CSA exam, is that patients will respond to empathic attitudes. Secondly, if the way you are approaching a consultation is not working, be prepared to change your approach – that is be truly patient-centred. Management plans not only need to take account of the current best practice, but, very importantly, also need to take into account individual patient factors – such as their fears, beliefs, or responsibilities (e.g. as carers). Finally, a reminder that time management is very important in allowing you to give enough attention to this section of the consultation, as it is most usually towards the end.

There is much more detail on how best to use Examiners' feedback statements in Chapter 6.

Exam-performance management

It has become apparent, in working with a range of GP registrars, and also with trainees in difficulty, that, for some people, exam-performance anxiety can be one of their main personal barriers to passing the CSA. Just as consultation skills can be learned, and practised, exam-performance management skills can also be learned and practised in your surgeries. There are also specific resources available to those who may need outside or specialist help. For example, barriers to success can be negative thinking, or self doubt, clouding the consultation and preventing you from truly hearing the patient.

Adapting neurolinguistic programming (NLP) resources to the GP consultation suggests tools such as identifying, challenging and replacing unhelpful thinking. For example, replace the fear, 'I will fail', with the fact that 'there is evidence my consultations are good' – as identified by trainer and patient satisfaction questionnaire feedback (Connolly/Pegasus, 2014).

Replace any worries you may have about any perceived weaknesses, with techniques to overcome these. For example, if you tend to speak very quickly, and this has caused patients difficulty in your consultations during training, then start the initial introduction deliberately calmly, slowly and with a smile. Focus on a warm tone, and try to avoid a very fast rate of speech, as this appears less empathic to patients. Don't forget, after each point you make, to leave a gap for the patient to respond. If any genuine misunderstandings occur during the interaction, don't be frightened to ask the patient to clarify, or check that they have taken in what you have said. Practise this through your consultations in the surgery.

'Act calmly'. Remember that your body language (e.g. sitting with shoulders hunched, looking down and not smiling, or even gritting your teeth!) has an impact both on your interaction and also your self confidence. The converse is also true – sitting in a relaxed physical posture, and calm breathing allows anxieties to fade into the background. This is a small part of how we can adapt our own behavioural responses to stress.

Care with non-verbal cues, such as being observant to the patient's body language, and also your own – such as comfortable eye contact, where often you and the patient mirror each other's eye contact – will be very effective.

In the CSA, at the 10-minute buzzer ending a consultation, clear all thoughts from your head. You really have no idea how many marks the examiner has just given you, so please use the time to gain information about the next case by reading the patient's records. It is essential to clear your head fully for the next case.

LEARNING POINT 4: Performance management tips

- Replace unhelpful, negative thinking with positive thoughts.
- Replace your concerns about your perceived weaknesses with tools to overcome them.
- Act calmly.
- Be aware of your own body language and non-verbal cues.
- When the buzzer ends the consultation in the CSA, clear your head for the next case.

In preparing yourself mentally for the exam, and in terms of housekeeping, you should decide how you intend to use the 2-minute break between patients. You should aim calmly to read the information in the patient records in the iPad, including whether any results, valuable past history or social history are available to you.

In addition, prior to taking the CSA, practise any relaxation or focusing techniques which work for you. In your day-to-day surgery, this can be done in the very short time that patients usually take to walk along the corridor to the consulting room, so that your mind is open and receptive to whatever the new patient is about to share with you. This can then be part of your preparation in the 2-minute gap between cases in the CSA. It may also be useful to practise beforehand how to apply this technique, in order to relax and refocus as quickly as possible in the CSA, if, for example, you have just had a very stressful consultation, such as an angry patient.

Conclusion

In conclusion, one of the theories in NLP is that we can learn techniques to achieve positive outcomes in our interactions with other people. This is surely the entire basis for us, as GPs, in looking at and practising consultation models and skills. This idea can, therefore, be expanded to practise stress management techniques in patient interactions, with a view to utilising it in clinical exam situations.

For the vast majority, such simple techniques, and the support of their trainer, are all that is needed. Some individuals may have identified that they need additional help with their anxieties around the exam. Cognitive behavioural therapy is one option, and a number of avenues exist for this, such as the 'Practitioner Health Programme' and also 'Mednet', which is provided by the professional support unit. Across the United Kingdom, your GP school would be able to signpost you to local resources. Please do not feel reticent about asking for such help, as all GP educators will be delighted to help solve a problem and even happier to see a good end result.

The aim of this section on exam-performance management is to help you to determine your goals for your CSA PDP, and to begin to prepare psychologically for the day of the exam, by practising and devising your coping strategies. We hope this will allow you to perform to the best of your ability and maximize your success.

Table of personal needs, following self assessment, with trainer input

My personal needs (based on possible perceived barriers)	My strategies to overcome and assist me in passing the CSA

Agreed CSA PDP – integrating learner and trainer conclusions.
This should also integrate feedback from any courses attended.

My agreed goals for target areas	Progress and comments

Tips and Hints – Getting Started

1.i Getting Started – Preparation for Taking the CSA

- Start your preparation early.
- Prepare to be challenged – and challenge yourself!
- Preparing for the CSA is about preparing for work as a real-life GP.
- Practise in the surgery and apply skills on real patients – in particular new patients.
- Use the resources of the practice – use all the team, use Out of Hours.
- It's a knowledge test too – consider taking a 'passmedicine.com' AKT refresher.
- Get exposed to stress early in the year – exposure leads to experience.
- Read around consultation skills.
- Read around the MRCGP curriculum.
- Hit the ground at Euston at a comfortable trot – if not running.
- Go in with a positive attitude.
- Work in small groups.
- Develop cases sampled from your day-to-day work – build on the case creation exercise in Chapter 5.
- Role-play being a candidate, being an examiner, being a patient.
- Stretch yourself by choosing cases with ethical dilemmas – reflect on the ethical dimension (see Chapter 4).
- Use video to reflect on your techniques.
- Use your trainer – joint surgeries/video.
- Show videos of challenging cases to your trainer/others.
- The COT is formative – competence in COT gives guidance about your readiness to take the CSA.
- Map the COT domains as appropriate and use the feedback statements to improve and groom you for the exam.
- You can always revert to the standard COT after the CSA.
- Try to do COTs with more than one trainer – a different perspective is often helpful.
- Do more than the minimum – the more you do, the more feedback you will get.
- When you are preparing for the exam in earnest, move on from COTs and just get your trainer to assess you on data-gathering, clinical management and interpersonal skills (plus a global comment).
- Put areas for improvement in the agreed actions in your run-up to the CSA (from your CSA PDP – see above).

The RCGP curriculum is daunting and ever changing. You need to be both current and to

- show aptitude for life-long learning
- check you have covered the curriculum adequately
- use your training needs assessments, inductions, reviews, tutorials as opportunities to assess and address your learning needs
- target your learning on current hot topics
- use the GP curriculum as your 'satnav' for learning throughout training
- review your e-portfolio: both the curriculum and eportfolio have been adopted into revalidation; you need them to navigate the territory 'towards the CSA and beyond'

We recommend 'RCGP – The Condensed Curriculum Guide' as an excellent overview and 'vade mecum'.

1.ii Getting Started – Materials to Use

Check out the RCGP Website – www.rcgp.org.uk – and follow the links to 'MRCGP Clinical Skills Assessment (CSA)'

There is a wealth of information here about the CSA, which is constantly updated. Here is a list of some of the materials available at the time of going to press –

- What is the clinical skills assessment (CSA)
- Format of the CSA
- Introduction to the CSA cases
- CSA walkthrough video
- Delivery of the CSA/use of iPads
- CSA booking procedure
- Dates of applications for CSA examinations and publication of results
- Apply for the CSA
- Declaring a disability or requesting special adjustments
- Preparing for the CSA
- Arrival and departure times
- Equipment required on the day
- Dress code
- Candidate briefing
- CSA marking
- Video recording
- CSA results and feedback

- CSA summary reports from September 2010 to December 2014
- Complaints, reviews and appeals

Use CSA case cards – RCGP Wessex
Watch and review 'A Guide to the CSA' – DVD exemplars – RCGP Wessex
Read 'The Condensed Curriculum' – pages 46–52
Target the MRCGP curriculum – especially 'Being a GP' core statement
We recommend that, to help prepare, you refer to the "Generic Indicators for targeted assessment domains" (http://www.rcgp.org.uk/training-exams/mrcgp-exams-overview/~/media/BD43B1D830F14793A92C505360F50D08.ashx)
This is a really useful tool for you and your trainer to use in video and observed surgeries, and to assist in small group work (see Chapter 5).

References

Connolly, R. (2014) Master practitioner in Neuro-Linguistic Programming + Pegasus website – www.nlp-now.co.uk/core_skills_syllabus.htm. Last accessed 28 August 2015.

CSA examiners' feedback statements. (2014) www.rcgp.org.uk. Last accessed 28 August 2015.

Eve, R. (2003) "PUNS and DENS: Discovering Learning Needs in General Practice". Oxford: Radcliffe Publishing Ltd. Luft J (*1* 961).

McKelvey, I. (2010) "The Consultaton Hill" Br J Gen Pract (BJGP) 60(576): 538–540.

Trafford, P. (2010) Retired associate director for trainees in difficulty London Deanery.

Chapter 2 **What you can learn from the 'patients'**

In Chapter 1 we focused on you, the candidate. This chapter is written from the perspective of the second element in the CSA – the simulated patients.

When you eventually come to take the CSA exam, and you are in your allocated 'surgery' at the RCGP Exam Centre in Euston reading through the notes on the iPad about the 13 'patients' about to come through the door, you will want to know that the role-players simulating those 'patients' are well prepared, and that they will give you every opportunity to show your consulting skills (Russell et al., 2011).

Who are these simulated 'patients'?

All CSA role-players are professional actors, but before they are allowed to embark upon the CSA itself, they have to attend a training session introducing them to the exam. We emphasise the gravity of the exam, the need for fairness and consistency, to ensure all candidates are given an equal opportunity to perform, and that the quality of their work will be continually assured by a regular direct observation or video monitoring process.

We discuss 'cueing' – not what actors normally expect as cueing – in the CSA, this means what information to give you, the candidate, and this may be done either verbally or non-verbally. The crucial message is that the role-player is your 'friend', who is there to point you to, and keep you on, the right path for the consultation. Everything that the 'patient' does or says is a cue. So, don't just listen to what the 'patient' is saying; watch the body language for cues as well. Even their appearance will be one of the first cues – the actors will 'look the part', they will be the appropriate age, ethnicity and physical appearance.

The CSA Exam: Maximizing your Success, First Edition. Rachel Roberts.

Companion Website: www.wiley.com\go\Roberts\CSAExam

Most importantly, they are instructed how to deal with you. If you use jargon or medical terminology which a lay person wouldn't understand, they will bat it back to you – 'I don't understand' – and the 26th and final candidate in the day will get exactly the same response, even though the actor may have had to do this 25 times already!

If you simply say 'I'd like to examine you', the actor is trained to say – 'What do you want to examine, what are you looking for' – so save yourself a few seconds and say exactly what physical examination you want to do and why.

LEARNING POINT 5: Verbalise your thoughts

Examiners can't read your mind! It is essential throughout the exam that you verbalise your thought process for the examiner to hear and mark.

For the actors, the most instructive part of the training is the session where they role play both parts – the 'patient' and then the doctor. You'll be gratified to hear that, when asked how it feels to play the doctor, the actors always say how hard it is and express admiration for the work that you do!

Calibration

The final session of the training for the actors prepares them for the 'Calibration Meeting' (Russell et al., 2011), which is the main means by which the 'patients' are standardised. The CSA takes place on three circuits, so every 'patient' is performed simultaneously by three role-players who are each paired with an examiner. At the Calibration Meeting prior to the exam on each day, the three examiners agree how the case will be marked, and the three role-players get the chance to practise the role, comparing and calibrating each other's portrayal of the 'patient' to attain consistency.

This is the actors' dress rehearsal and each will have a run-through at the meeting. They will have received their Case Briefing Notes (two or three A4 pages of background information about the patient) about a week before the day of the exam. The only part of the case which is actually scripted is the opening statement, and the wording of this, the tone in which it is delivered, and the accompanying body language will be practised by each actor at the start and end of the meeting. At the beginning of each consultation, the 'patient' knocks, enters and sets the tone for the next 10 minutes by giving the opening statement exactly as worded and in the calibrated manner.

It is of paramount importance that all three role-players have the chance during the meeting to practise their role properly, and to learn from observing each other's performance. The examiners will also contribute their experience of patients seen in their surgeries with problems similar to the case being prepared. Thus, in order to achieve consistency and standardisation in the way the three actors portray the same case, agreement must be reached by all at the Calibration Meeting on the crucial elements – not just the delivery of the opening statement, but also the demeanour of the 'patient' and, crucially, cueing.

The cueing of information to the candidate (i.e. what information to give, how and when) is case-specific, but each Case Briefing Notes for the actors contains answers to be given to questions the typical candidate will ask (see the CSA-type case exemplars in Part 2). At the Calibration Meeting, decisions will be made as to how much information to give at each stage of the consultation – for example, how to respond to open questions or the typical 'Tell me more ... '

Because the level of assertiveness or anxiety to be projected by all three actors must be consistent if the exam is to be fair, it is vital that the role-players observe each other's run-through and adapt their own performance, where necessary, in order to standardise the personality, tone of voice and non-verbal cues.

Where a case involves actual physical examination, each of the role-players will be examined by the GP assessors during the Calibration Meeting. This is firstly to ensure that the actors have no potentially confusing signs or medical conditions which could affect the candidate's diagnosis. Secondly, it acts as a reassurance to the actors if during the day a candidate makes a false diagnosis. The role-players may be asked to mimic physical findings – for example a painful arc of shoulder movement – and the assessors will explain how to react to the physical examination, both physically and verbally. Where exactly is the site of the pain? What level of pain is it? Does the problem affect the 'patient' in other ways – for example walking, sitting?

What do the role-players think about the CSA exam?

Much research has been undertaken with the simulated 'patients', for example to discover what they think of the CSA exam itself, and what, in their eyes, makes a good candidate (Russell et al., 2012). Actual comments from the research are shown below in italics.

The actors are very aware just how important the CSA is, and of their responsibilities in ensuring a fair and reliable exam for all. In general, they think that the CSA is a fair test and about as realistic as it could be. They are proud of their part in that – '*We have an enabling role*' – allowing candidates to show their consulting capabilities.

However, they also know that once the opening statement is given, what happens next depends entirely on you, the candidate. '*We know we've got to get from A to B, but if they don't give you the triggers, I can't go*'. The flow of the consultation depends on the questions you ask and on your behaviour – '*my responses change because of the way the GP deals with me – my reactions and emotions change*'.

So, what makes a good consulter – according to the actors?

The very best, patient-centred doctors understand the impact the particular problem is having on that 'patient' – for example with their family, or at work. They are able to enter the 'patient's' life-world and see issues of health and illness from a patient's perspective. '*They were responding to my cues and joining in and seeing my frustrations. They understood the impact it was having*'. Such GPs are then able to select from a range of consulting styles and skills to be able to deal with those issues.

LEARNING POINT 6: Active listening [1]
As well as just listening, *your* body language, eye contact and demeanour are all essential in making the patient want to talk and open up to you.

The way you encourage dialogue by the use of your body language is crucial. A good consulter will '*nod and agree, and encourage you, and be more positive with the body language, eye contact … suddenly there's this natural sense of interest, and my whole demeanour changes towards them*'. And that positive reaction starts to form within the first few seconds, based on both verbal and non-verbal aspects – the quality of the welcome (e.g. standing to greet the patient), introductions, eye contact, smiling and so on.

LEARNING POINT 7: Active listening [2]
Remember that the role-player has been primed to 'cue' you, so listen to what you are being told and watch for non-verbal cues. For the first minute or so of the consultation try to say as little as possible yourself, just using positive body language and open questions or phrases to encourage the 'patient' to open up to you.

LEARNING POINT 8: Active listening [3]
'Tell me more' may simply lead to the 'patient' replying 'What do you want to know?' So try to make the question more specific – for example 'Tell me when they (headaches) start'.

LEARNING POINT 9: Active listening [4]
Listen and reflect explicitly – 'You said earlier ... '; 'Did I hear you say ... '

Asking the right questions

Questions, designed to elicit the patient's Ideas, Concerns and Expectations, are a valuable questioning tool, but they must only be used when relevant and appropriate – and certainly not by rote! '*I've got to be caring here, I've got to ask this question here ... It's as if they're thinking, 'I'm going to ask this, irrespective of what you've just said, this is how I want to move it on' – and that's different from somebody who is genuinely interested*'.

So, for example, if the opening statement makes absolutely clear the nature and gravity of the situation which the 'patient' wants to be dealt with, it is inappropriate to ask 'What were you hoping we might do today?'

There are few cases where there is a hidden agenda. If the 'patient' is making good eye contact, talking normally with open body language and friendly demeanour, there is unlikely to be a hidden agenda. So, in such instances, the repetition of the question – 'Is there anything else?' – is not usually necessary once the patient has said 'No'. Cues and hints which are not immediately obvious and take a bit more skill and experience to reveal is NOT the same as 'hidden'!

LEARNING POINT 10: Hidden agendas
If there *is* a hidden agenda, the clues for you will usually be in the body language, lack of eye contact, slow or distracted speech.

Similarly, you should also only question about smoking, alcohol and so on if it is actually relevant to the case.

According to the research, however, many actors hate being asked – Did you have any thoughts about what it might be?' – usually responding – 'No, you're the doctor, you tell me!' In our opinion, however, they are wrong to dismiss the question, and a follow-up such as – 'It's just that some people come with their theories' – can often elicit further, valuable information.

LEARNING POINT 11: Why candidates may fail on interpersonal skills

A candidate who fails on interpersonal skills

- Does not use positive body language and eye contact to encourage the patient to talk
- Does not listen and then respond to what the patient is saying
- Does not respond to cues – verbal or non-verbal – given by the patient
- Shows a lack of genuine interest by talking over or lecturing the patient
- Is not genuinely empathetic towards the patient
- Does not interact with the patient as in a proper conversation
- Does not involve the patient in the diagnosis or clinical management
- Ticks the boxes of his/her own agenda, asking questions by rote, no matter what the patient is saying
- Uses Social, Psycho-social, Ideas, Concerns and Expectations (SPICE) questions insensitively and inappropriately
- Does not get to the point, or fails to comprehend the patient's agenda
- Does not understand the impact of the problem on the patient's life, family, work and so on
- Offers leaflets, not explanations (examiners cannot mark leaflets!)

Time management

At the start of the data-gathering phase remember that in the CSA you will never have met any of the 'patients', so spend the first few minutes of the consultation listening to the patient's agenda and finding out about their *S*ocial and *P*sycho-social background and *ICE* by asking open questions. We refer to this methodology as 'SPICE'.

Closed questions will then be needed to do the 'doctor-centred' bit – that is checking on symptoms, red-flags and eliminating serious illness.

LEARNING POINT 12: Structure your consultation

You need to have a clear structure in mind for your consultation, and to remember to include the 'patient' by sharing ideas, options and decisions throughout.

You will also need to decide if you need to do a physical examination. On most exam days three to four cases will entail some form of a physical examination.

LEARNING POINT 13: Physical examination 1

If it is appropriate to examine on a day-to-day basis in your surgery, then it is appropriate to do so in the CSA – and to do it properly because your technique will be assessed!

LEARNING POINT 14: Physical examination 2

Think about the scenarios entailing actual physical examination – joints, for example – which are likely to occur in the CSA, and watch videos of good practice for such examinations.

In some cases, it is perfectly appropriate for a physical examination to be done, but the case-writers know that there is not enough time for that within the 10 minutes of the CSA exam. In these circumstances, once you have explained what you are going to examine and what you are looking for, the examiner will give you an 'asset' – that is the results of your examination. This may be done with a card or photo, or simply verbally by the examiner.

After 5 or 6 minutes of data-gathering and history-taking, you should be getting on to the development of your management plan. This must be evidence-based and include appropriate follow-up and inclusion of the patient in the decision making.

LEARNING POINT 15: Timing the consultation

Don't spend too much time on the data-gathering to the detriment of management! Many candidates fail because of an inadequate or inappropriate management plan.

'Patient' diversity

Virtually any patient or situation which GPs encounter in their surgeries is feasible in the CSA, so you need to think about diversity and how it might affect your consultation. How, for example, will you deal with a blind patient? Or one who is profoundly deaf? How will you consult with both a parent and a child in the room? Or with a carer who comes along with his or her patient?

LEARNING POINT 16: Gender balance
Half of each day's CSA cases will be male, the other half female. How much exposure do you get in your day-to-day surgery dealing with both genders? Male trainees, for example, often don't see the gynaecology or contraception cases.

LEARNING POINT 17: The 'angry patient' 1
One of the cases you encounter in the CSA may involve an 'angry patient'. The crucial thing to remember here is that you have never met the person before, so they can never actually be angry at you – but at some incident. Apologising *for the situation the person finds themselves in* as early as possible in the consultation (without making judgements or taking sides) will diffuse much of the anger.

LEARNING POINT 18: The 'angry patient' 2
Remember to keep calm, not to mirror the angry person's speech patterns, tone of voice or body language. Such cases are always difficult, but remind yourself that everyone doing the exam on that day will also have to deal with it and will find it equally hard.

And, finally, remember …

Patient-centredness is the gold standard, but this does not mean letting the patient talk all the time, or necessarily getting what they want, if it's inappropriate. You are the doctor and there are roles for doctor and patient. You have the professional expertise which the patients are seeking for their problems.

So, when the buzzer goes at the CSA exam and that first 'patient' walks through the door, remember that (s)he is there to enable you to perform at your best and to demonstrate that professional expertise.

The role-player is your 'friend' and has been carefully trained to 'cue' you. So, listen carefully and watch the body language!

Tips and Hints – The Consultation

2.i Practise, Practise, Practise!

- Get the right habits from the start.
- Don't ever practise in one way when you are unobserved in the surgery, and in a different way if the video is on, if your trainer is observing the consultation, or if you are in the CSA exam.
- Do it how you normally do it – and start doing it early. It shows if you haven't had enough – or the right – experience.
- Practise active listening – monitoring your own body language and non-verbal behaviours.
- Reflect on consultations that go well, and, when they don't go well, ask yourself why they don't. Are there doctor-factors you can address – for example being stressed yourself?
- Practise giving and receiving feedback – what helps?
- Assume in the CSA that you are in a normal surgery with usual facilities.
- Practise running through your management plans with your trainer.
- Get good with examination/especially joints.
- Use the physical examination part of the consultation as a pivot point.
- Look at the exam as an excuse to learn skills and techniques that will help you enjoy your professional life and help patients more.
- Everyone is putting on a performance, practise playing your part genuinely.
- Get inside the examiner's head.
- Reflect on and use the positive feedback statements (Chapter 6).

2.ii Language

- Use SPICE questions to investigate the patient's psycho-social background – it may take you to the nub (but ensure they are appropriate).
- Avoid mechanistic CSA exam jargon (e.g. '*Is it OK if I ask you a few specific questions*').
- Find alternatives to '*Tell me more*' being more specific.
- Use simple reflections – '*You mentioned earlier...*'
- Use the patient record if appropriate – '*It says here that …*'
- Don't recite the obvious.

- Get fluent in the majority of clinical areas.
- Use patient information leaflets to learn how to explain medical conditions in patient-friendly, lay language.
- Practise different consultation techniques so that you can change tack if necessary should the consultation be going awry.
- Only ask about alcohol and smoking if relevant.
- Be aware of culturally appropriate use of language and space – be professional.

2.iii Time Management

- Get used to consulting in 10 minutes.
- Structure your consultations – roughly 5–6 minutes taking the history and examining, then move to management.
- Get used to your internal body clock telling when 5 minutes have passed.
- Use good general consulting skills – summarise, screen, safety-net.
- Avoid repetition – listen and note.
- Don't waste time searching for a hidden agenda which isn't there.
- In the CSA itself, you'll be keeping your eye on the count-up clock on the wall.
- To prepare for this, have a clock on a shelf behind the patients in your surgery.
- Set up a count-up clock on your computer screen.
- Use your analysis of videos to identify where you have potential to improve time management.
- You need to be able to prioritise, deal with the unexpected, be flexible to the needs of the patient and the context.

2.iv Consultations to Cover

- See lots of patients – practise, practise, practise.
- Accept responsibility for following patients.
- Worry if you have not collected a cohort of patients who see you more regularly.
- Help with result and mail processing.
- Help with repeat prescribing.
- Question processes and things you don't understand – this will help you learn.
- OOH is a good place to learn.
- Do telephone consultations.
- Go on difficult visits.
- Attend chronic disease management clinics.
- Get real multi-source feedback – small groups, OOH supervisor.

- Be knowledgeable – keep a subscription to 'passmedicine.com'.
- Sit a paper or two in the weeks before doing the CSA

Cover the Right Areas

- Straightforward clinical situations requiring a physical examination.
- Emotionally charged situations (e.g. anger, grief).
- Complex clinical problems and *Ethical Dilemmas* – (Chapter 4) – consider impact on work/driving.
- Undifferentiated patient presentations (multiple morbidity, unclear diagnoses).
- Practise your clinical management in the surgery as much as you can.
- A good and credible management plan will depend on getting the right differential diagnosis – use Case Cards to practise.
- Don't forget everyday illnesses.
- Patient diversity (ethnicity, disability).
- Professional behaviour, for example colleagues.
- Remember the CSA is like a normal surgery, but where every patient is a new patient to you.
- Ask your reception team to fit new patients in with you – it's even better if they consent to be videoed.

Know Your Blind Spots

- Some candidates fall down because they have clearly not encountered some situations in their practices.
- Avoid going for easy visits or easy consultations in the OOH centre, but use them to broaden your experience.
- Consider a short attachment to a different kind of practice if you feel your experience is limited for example rural, inner city.
- If you are a male registrar with a male trainer, then be aware of possible blind spots in womens' health and vice versa.
- Be cool with sexual health – be able to take a sexual health history without giggling.

At its core, general practice and the CSA are about effective consulting – learn how to consult effectively
There are a plethora of courses to choose from

- Medical schools, training programmes and deaneries provide consultation skills courses at early stages of training.

- It is well worth refreshing your approach to consultation skills regularly as part of your preparation for the exam, as well as getting detailed feedback from your trainer. Video analysis may be especially powerful.
- With regard to the CSA specifically, feedback suggests that courses which include a simulated exam are highly valued by candidates. You may wish to take advantage of one of the courses based at Euston Square, the new 'home', of the College. These courses usually include a tour of the exam centre – 'The Euston Square GP practice' – which is likewise highly valued by delegates and can help you feel more at home when your return for your exam. There are virtual tours available online, but there is nothing quite such as the bricks, concrete and Victorian tile work of *your* College – it's well worth a visit, and the College enjoys welcoming AiTs to its 'home'.

References

Russell, D., Simpson, R., Rendel, S. (2011) "Standardisation of role players for the Clinical Skills Assessment of the MRCGP" Educ Primary Care 22 (3): 166–170.

Russell, D., Etherington, C., Hawthorne, K. (2012) "How can simulated patients' experiences suggest ways to improve candidate performance in the CSA?" Educ Primary Care 23 (6): 391–398.

Chapter 3 **What to expect in the CSA**

The previous two chapters focused mainly on you, the candidate, and the simulated patients. The aim in this chapter is to complete the triangle of elements involved in preparation for the CSA – the Candidate, the Simulated Patient and the Assessment itself, by helping you to become familiar with the framework of the exam itself, the practical elements and what is expected of you. This should help you prepare sufficiently and feel more comfortable and 'at home' on the day of your exam.

'Being a general practitioner'

Think back to why and when you first wanted to be a GP. This test is about whether you can demonstrate to your peers that you can be. It is about 'Being a GP', a test of performance in relation to your knowledge, skills and attitudes, underpinned by your experience. So revisit the RCGP core curriculum statement – 'Being a GP'.

Preparing for the exam

In the process of preparing for and taking the CSA, you should expect to acquire the knowledge, skills and attitudes that will help you enjoy examination success and RCGP membership – but most importantly, that will equip you for your life as a GP. Again we urge you be aware of your personal barriers – but see the opportunities for professional development and enhanced job satisfaction that come from performing well as a GP. In short, expect a test that tests what is expected of you.

The CSA Exam: Maximizing your Success, First Edition. Rachel Roberts.

Companion Website: www.wiley.com\go\Roberts\CSAExam

A definition of the CSA

The CSA has been defined as a test of ability under controlled conditions to '*integrate and apply appropriate clinical professional communication and practical skills in general practice*'. It is worth dissecting and considering this definition.

'*Integrate*' means you need to do it all together FLUENTLY in a seamless consultation. The whole is more than the sum of the parts. A common refrain on CSA courses is '*practise all the skills, all the time*'.

'*Appropriate*' means you need to do it in the context of the patient's presentation, in general practice. This is to say you should adopt an approach that takes into account the needs and setting of the individual patient. This is an RCGP exam and it is, therefore, wise to remember the *triaxial* RCGP model of the consultation (1972), that is to consider the *Medical Psychological* and *Social* aspects of each and every consultation.

'*Clinical*' means you need to demonstrate an awareness of current accepted clinical norms and best practice: efficient and effective medicine, evidence-based practice, knowledge of therapeutic options and their limitations.

'*Professional*' means you need to display the behaviour and attitudes of a doctor as described in GMC guidance which provides the ethical underpinning to professional training and revalidation – making the 'best care of your patient your first concern', showing courtesy and respect for your patients, but working within personal and system resources including relationships, and being aware of your 'duties as a doctor'.

'*Communication*' is a key element involving listening, facilitating, explaining, conveying meaning, checking, understanding, and cultural sensitivity: ability to deal with anger and conflict, and to convey bad news.

'*Practical*' means you need to display a pragmatic and capable approach in history-taking, physical examination, time management, use of instruments and scarce NHS resources, and to show technical proficiency.

In summary you need to apply the correct, evidence-based knowledge at the correct time in the best way.

LEARNING POINT 19: Be yourself!

In the CSA you should be your normal, doctoring self. The CSA is simply examining good general practice, so don't try to act any differently from the way you are on a day-to-day basis, or – put another way – act the way you do in the CSA in your normal life as a GP, and you won't go wrong.

How the exam is structured

The exam comprises a circuit of 13 'stations' designed to give each candidate the same series of testing consultations. The intention is to recreate a standardised environment that approximates to a challenging morning or afternoon in general practice. You are extremely *unlikely* to see nothing but sore throats and depression, or to have the feeling that things always come in threes! You are very *likely* to be tested on a broad range of knowledge, skills and attitudes referenced to the curriculum. So the best preparation is to know your territory, to know your blind spots and get practice on them, and generally to gain plenty of GP experience.

In essence, the assessment comprises 13 snapshots *building a picture* of you as a GP from a 'palette' of carefully selected, simulated patient scenarios, anchored in the curriculum from the case bank (see below). You will be assessed by 13 trained, professional peers independently across three skills domains (data-gathering, clinical management and interpersonal skills, IPS). The patients are played by 13 trained, professional role-players as has been described in Chapter 2.

Timing

You stay put as you normally would in surgery, and the patients come to you. The cases are designed to be do-able in 10 minutes, the current, typical UK consultation time, and for you to be able to maximize your scores in all three marked domains in that time. At one level, it is a test of your ability to time-manage (organisational skills). Importantly, you get at least 2 minutes between 'patients' to prepare ('housekeep') for the next case (you get more before the first case), and there is a coffee break of 10–15 minutes in the middle of your surgery. Thus, it is worth remembering that the cases are at least 12 minutes long and you should be thinking of them this way.

LEARNING POINT 20: Read the patient records

It is good practice to spend 2 minutes looking at the summary patient records – medications and last consultation, relevant recent results, correspondence (the kind of information generally gleaned from good housekeeping). In this sense, you are already gathering data and increasing your likelihood of having an efficient and effective consultation and setting the tone of your greeting – a great habit to get into not just for the CSA but also for your life as a GP.

It is the only surgery you will ever have where the patient dutifully gets up and walks out when a 10-minute buzzer sounds! You might consider speaking to your trainer about how best to 'simulate the simulation'. One method is to set up an appointment schedule based on the CSA timings – that is a basic template of 13 patients in 13 × 10 minute appointments, perhaps with 2-minute catch-up slot in between and a 10-minute break.

LEARNING POINT 21: A CSA-style appointments schedule template

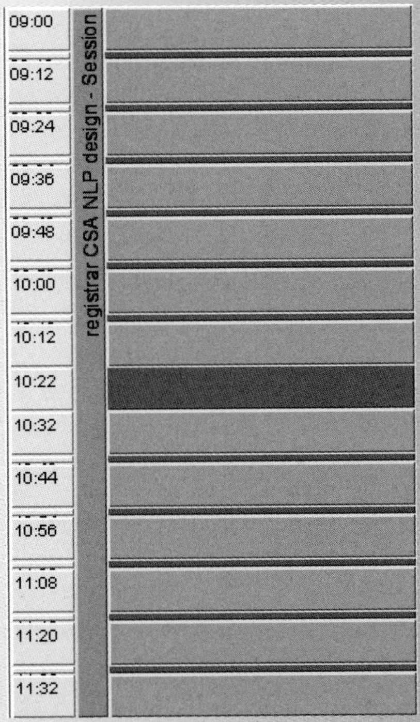

Setting the scene

There will be a telephone on the desk. Your palette may include a telephone case. If it rings, answer it! You may have heard the story of a candidate who in the early days of the CSA, true to the spirit of the exam, actually dialled 999 for a very sick patient and got directly connected to the emergency services! This glitch has now been corrected!

Likewise, your palette may include a home visit. If this is the case, a 'marshal' will come and fetch you to take you to the 'home visit' room. No car or driving licence is required in this instance!

There is no computer on the desk, no need to code entries or be distracted by Quality and Outcomes Framework (QOF) point flags. This is not to say being ignorant of QOF and its evidenced-based focus is a good thing. Indeed, demonstrating awareness of the QOF agenda by routine reference to smoking and smoking cessation, where appropriate, may be good practice, but rote-learned, mechanical lecturing is unlikely to score you additional marks. The 'quality outcome' to go for in the CSA is a high-quality, rounded consultation (with perhaps a bit of QOF on the side for good measure). 'Master Chef' rather than 'Boil in the Bag'.

When with patients, it is worth practising minimising your use of the computer. New patients are ideal for this purpose. They often have no, or scant records, and you have no computer to distract you from human interaction.

It may be stating the obvious to say you will be 'out of your comfort zone in the CSA'; unfamiliar surroundings, no comfort blanket PC to play with or Internet to refer to, potentially more challenging and risky cases. So it's worth practising in environments and situations that simulate the simulation – ask to see new patients and 'walk-ins' in the practice, make the most of your Out of Hours sessions and supervision. Visit the exam centre if you can.

Who are the examiners?

The examiners panel comprises a heterogeneous group of upwards of 240 practising GPs 'in good standing'. This panel size is maintained for statistical and logistical purposes and to ensure enough examiners are available to cover every diet. Examiners come in all shapes, sizes, ages, colours, creeds, and gender orientations. Protected characteristics are reflected in the composition of the panel, and all examiners have regular equality and diversity training. Not all trainers are educationalists, although many are. They have to take the AKT and attend training seminars before being accepted on to the panel. They also continue to be trained on the job and attend a compulsory, annual training conference.

LEARNING POINT 22: Observers

Don't be alarmed if, during your CSA exam, more than one apparent 'assessor' enters the room. There are often 'occasional others'. These may include

Quality Assurance personnel who are monitoring the role-players, or visiting dignitaries, lay observers, observers from other colleges, or interested bodies such as the Care Quality Commission (CQC) and GP schools representatives.

So how does it all run on the day?

You will be allocated a morning or an afternoon session. The afternoon candidates are 'quarantined' over lunch time to prevent 'cross contamination' or communication. No lunch is provided to afternoon candidates, so eat first.

Arrive in good time and enter via the candidates' entrance on Euston Road. If you are coming from Euston mainline Rail Station or from the Victoria/Northern underground lines, you need to cross Melton Street and walk about 100 yards west/to the right up Euston Road. If you are coming from Euston Square Underground station (Circle/Metropolitan lines), you need to exit on the north side, turn left and walk 100 yards east down Euston road towards the mainline Rail Station.

On arrival at the Examination Centre, you will need to show your identification (Driver's Licence/passport/NHS photo ID) – and you will receive a candidate's pass. There are modest lockers for you to store luggage.

You will need a basic diagnostic kit: stethoscope, torches, sphygmomanometer, your ophthalmoscope/auriscope and patella hammer. It is best to bring your own basic examining equipment which you are comfortable with. You also need to know and show how to use them! A definitive list is given on the College CSA website. Less usual instruments (e.g. tuning fork) or those needing to be sterile (e.g. tongue depressors) will be provided. Other materials may also be provided in your pack on the desk – (e.g. peak flow/growth chart).

Only a paper BNF is allowed. This can be tabbed for ease of reference but cannot be annotated or highlighted (it will be checked by the floor marshal before the exam). No other reference materials are allowed. PDAs and mobile phones must be switched off and left outside the exam circuit.

Any disabilities should be notified beforehand to the Exams department at the College so that appropriate provision can be made.

All this information will be rehearsed and repeated in your orientation meeting with the lead marshal for the day. It is also all available to read in detail on the RCGP CSA exam website. The marshals are all very experienced and generally good-humoured examiners. They are there to make the exam run smoothly for you and the examination team, and are supported and aided by dedicated members of the examination administration team who likewise are there to help with practicalities and stage management.

During this initial briefing, you will be given all the usual advice about fire drills, toilets, cautions, cheating and copyright, and any special on-the-day potential issues (e.g. noise or replacement role-players who may not 'look the part' because the original actor had to be replaced). You will also be drilled on the use of iPads. After some initial glitches, these now seem to be running smoothly. They are popular with candidates – and even the examiners are getting used to them!

Fire drills do happen – it is testimony to the efficiency of the examination and to the dedication and professionalism of all participants in the endeavour that these seem to pass off without a hitch – the centre is evacuated, and when the 'All Clear' sounds, everyone returns to the exam corridors and the cases restart like clockwork. (Any interrupted cases start again from the beginning.)

There are usually three parallel circuits running simultaneously – red, blue and purple – and you will be allocated to one of these. At the end of the briefing, you will be conducted to your circuit and room. In order to comply with E&D recommendations, only your GMC number appears on the door. Check that this number is correct. Your iPad should be logged on for you already – again check your details are correct. The phone on the desk will be functioning for exam purposes only – sadly you can't dial out of the building or 'phone a friend'. Likewise, the iPad can only be used for exam functions.

Every room has a fisheye camera and video and sound recording which is used for QA and training purposes.

The most unusual feature of the consultation room is the count-up timer clock which will be over the patient's left shoulder – visible to you and the examiner, but not to the patient.

LEARNING POINT 23: Time-keeping

It is worth recreating the time-up clock in your own consulting room to give yourself a feel for exam conditions, and it will help you manage consultation time more effectively. By getting a 'feel' for what a 5-minute span is like, you will know when to start to move into the clinical management stage of a 10-minute consultation.

You have may have up to 10 minutes in your room before the exam proper starts. During this time, you can read through the notes of your cases on the iPad, that is start data-gathering! This is a great habit to learn and apply in everyday practice.

For the exam, it is good to note if and when you have a telephone case or a home visit (you will not have both). In the final countdown to the start of the exam, it is best to focus on the patient notes of your first case; and to remember to use the precious time between cases to do the same for each upcoming case.

Read the notes!

This is so important. There is information which you need to conduct the consultation well, and it is gifted to you. Whether it is a face-to-face or third-party consultation, telephone triage or home visit, the patient record may contain clues about the patient's problem. The records are deliberately not a full medical history in order to avoid red herrings. More or less information may be significant in telling you that the patient attends frequently or rarely. A recent consultation with the nurse may give you useful information from tests, such as an ECG or spirometry (such information may help you target physical examination appropriately), or there may be a letter from a relative or consultant. This information is there for a reason – it's your first cue – yet amazingly, some candidates don't appear to make use of the records at all! Please don't be one of them.

LEARNING POINT 24: Data-gathering
The first 'cue' you get about each patient in the CSA is the information written in the patient records. So start your data-gathering for each case as soon as possible.

When the buzzer sounds, the count-up clock starts, there will be a knock on the door, or the phone will ring (unless you are starting with a home visit before surgery!) … and you're away.

So now what happens?

The 'patient' will usually knock on the door and is in role from the start. The 'patient'/role-player will interact with you just as a normal patient would, while following the briefing which they have been given and directions agreed with examiners as to how to pitch their emotional level. You should greet them as appropriate – your response may be tempered by information you have gleaned from the records. There are times when the hearty leap from the chair and clubbable handshake may be completely inappropriate. A friendly, helpful but neutral professional greeting, stating your name and asking how you can help, is safest – but be informed by your assessment of the records and the 'patient's' body language and verbal or non-verbal communication (eye contact, tone of voice, etc.– all of which will have been carefully calibrated and rehearsed, as explained in Chapter 2).

The only scripted element of the 'patient's' role is the opening statement, which may be embellished by body language or props. Listen to it. They won't tell you everything all at once and may not necessarily respond generously to entreaties such as '*tell me more*', so you will have to use direct and open questions to get all the information that you need.

Ignore the examiners

The examiners are only there to watch. They *might* occasionally intervene – generally later in the consultation – to provide examination findings, to hand you a card with findings, or to tell you that a particular examination (e.g. blood pressure) is not necessary on this occasion or is '*normal*'. This, however, will only happen if it has been agreed in the course of calibrating the case and at the examiner's discretion.

What kind of cases will I see?

The cases are all written by examiners and are based on their actual experience in practice. They are carefully blueprinted against the curriculum, and tested and piloted before being implemented in the exam itself. They present challenges that you may meet in any morning or afternoon surgery (see our sample cases in Part 2).

There is already a case bank of over 700 and it is growing. They are not rare or extraordinary cases, although some may be uncommon in practice in order to test your recognition of an urgent or rarer situation.

There are no trick questions or concealed agendas, although in some cases the patient has a problem that needs to be elicited by good consultation skills, for example attention to body language and non-verbal cues.

Some cases are undifferentiated, meaning that there is no clear diagnosis, and you have to proceed on the basis of probabilities and risk. Don't feel you have necessarily missed the 'answer', there may simply not be one – just like everyday general practice. If you are well experienced in general practice, this will feel and be straightforward.

In summary, you will be presented with a wide range of consultation challenges from general practice, which may present in the form of emergency, acute or chronic conditions, preventive medicine or service requests; conditions that are common, or less common conditions that may be serious.

A recent addition is the advent of children (no younger than 8 years old) attending with a parent.

At least one paediatric case is tested in each CSA exam circuit. However, since the CSA commenced in 2007, consultations about children below 13 years old were done by the parent alone, who, for example comes in to talk about a child left at home, or consults via telephone triage (14- to 15-year-old children may have been portrayed by role-players aged 16 or more, who look younger than their years).

In order to improve the reality of the exam, and to test different forms of consultation techniques, the RCGP researched using real children acting as 'patients'.

After lengthy trialling how best to calibrate child actors, cases involving children aged approximately 8 years or above, who come with their parents to the consultation, were introduced in 2013 and have now become a regular feature of exam diets, testing a candidate's ability to consult with two people in the room and with a young person.

We have included three paediatric cases in the sample cases in the Part 2 to reflect this addition and to enable you to practise such consultations.

So the 'patients' in the exam can be of *any* age, sex, social class, ethnic origin, occupation or level of intelligence. There are, of course, some limitations to what can be simulated. Parents may consult on behalf of very young children, carers consulting on behalf of the elderly infirm may involve a telephone call. There is (we hope) nothing actually physically wrong with the role-players themselves, so for fixed physical signs pictures and photos are used.

The exam is constantly evolving to improve its face validity for real-life practice.

The CSA has been negatively described as 'a surgery from hell'. It is not really helpful to approach it with this mindset. Expect it to be appropriately challenging. It will be more so in some cases than others; it is meant to be a challenge, after all. General Practice is challenging and getting more so. Ask yourself if you are up to it yet? Are you ready? Taking any of the exams before you are ready and have had sufficient experience is an expensive way to practice for it, both financially and in terms of your morale, but don't delay sitting it if you are good enough and ready.

See enough cases in day-to-day practice; fundamentally the CSA is a test of this experience.

So what is expected of me now?

Do what you do best! Continue integrating and applying your knowledge, skills and attitudes. In reality you are doing all the skills, all the time, to a varying extent and to a varying level of competence in every consultation you do. As you prepare for the CSA, you need to optimise your demonstration of this to the highest possible level. It is helpful perhaps to think of a 'CSA model consultation' (see illustration).

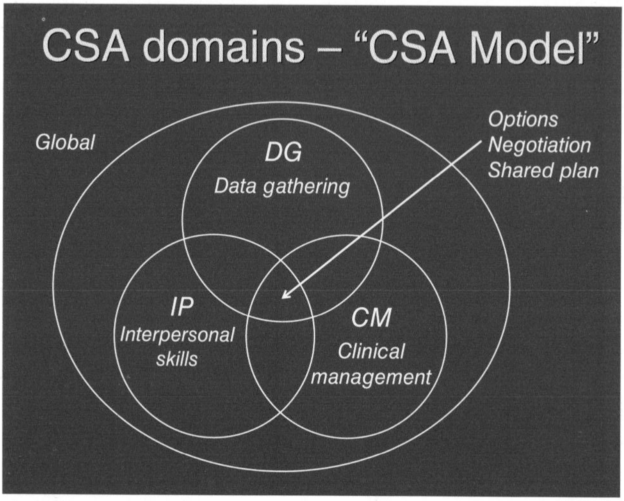

Create a global Impression

Think about your consultations globally. Adopt an organised approach, 'get to the nub', recognising dilemmas and using time effectively. 'Practise, practise, practise'.

Data-gathering (DG)

As has been emphasised, this phase begins before the consultation with *reading the notes* about the 'patient'. Doing this may inform your greeting and interpersonal interactions as well as help target your initial history taking and streamline your approach to clinical management.

Remember that this is a general practice consultation, so it doesn't require comprehensive 'clerking' of the 'patient'. It needs to be focused on their presenting complaint; to do this you need to listen and encourage the 'patient' to tell their *story*.

Closed questions are needed to support and exclude different possibilities. Open questions are needed to elicit background, social and psychological factors and to contextualise the presentation. You should remember to enquire for social and occupational history – whether given or not – and refer to it, if relevant, for example for a patient with cough or chest pains '*I can see in your notes that you smoke – how much do you smoke?'* demonstrates good data-gathering skills … and signals to the examiner that you have read the notes.

In doing a physical examination, the examiner wants to see what you choose to do and how you do it. Can you examine competently and recognise and act on clinical signs? Appropriate physical examination is expected and is marked. You have to decide whether to do an examination and which one(s) to do. Be guided by the history and be aware that there is a time limit of 10 minutes for the consultation; so time spent doing an examination may displace other more important elements of the consultation, thereby losing you marks. If you do an examination, do it properly; you will not score marks if your technique is poor and would miss an abnormal sign. Remember stage management as much as the technical intricacies. Look and sound as if you have done it before, ask about comfort and chaperoning. If intimate examination is indicated, ask (but don't persist if the patient declines). Show that you know how to hold lights and use instruments. It is fine to carry on chatting and relaxing the patient while being caring and courteous. Gain marks on your technique and courtesy – show 'professionalism'.

You can ask patients to remove clothes – listening through a shirt will not impress the examiner! Depending on how the case has been calibrated, the examiner may or may not intervene to say, for example 'the rest of the examination is normal'. You may or may not be given a card with the findings – do not appear to 'expect' this, however, by turning hopefully to the examiner.

LEARNING POINT 25: The pivot point

In terms of exam technique, utilising the examination phase of a case as a *pivot point* to move on from the Data-Gathering phase into the Clinical Management phase may be helpful. While the patient is getting themselves back together is a good time for you to confidently open up a discussion about diagnosis and management – for example

'Did you have any thoughts about what is going on here and what we might do about it?' ['not really, doctor'] … 'having listened to what you have said, and examined you carefully, what I think is … what do you think?'

Clinical management (CM)

The phases in a good consultation intersect or 'morph' into each other. Explaining the likely problem and/or diagnosis leads into a consideration of effective and safe treatment options. Clear and correct explanations are important not only as a clinical skill, but they also tell us about your problem-solving abilities – you are giving the examiner your assessment of the problem, as well as explaining it to the 'patient'. The sufficiently practised doctor will do this with fluency in most situations. Your management needs to be effective and safe. This is quality assurance for the public that you are fit for independent practice. Appropriate use of tests, drugs and referral is important. You need to balance the needs of the patient with the efficacy, cost and availability of the intervention. Brain scans, for example, are not first line for tension headache in UK practice – but containing and managing the expectation that one is needed, maintaining an ongoing, working relationship with the patient and safety-netting appropriately are key GP skills.

The examiner may need to know that you can recognise an emergency and act safely when presented with potentially serious situations, that you can weigh up risk and explain it to patients, and that you can modify your management to take account of co-morbidity and, where relevant, promote a healthy lifestyle.

Follow-up arrangements should be related to the practical needs of the situation and convey personal commitment by the doctor. Time is a great healer and diagnostic tool – use it wisely. You may not tell every patient in real life to come back for review but you need to demonstrate appropriate safety-netting for patients and have regard for continuity of care – a mantra of the RCGP.

LEARNING POINT 26: Clinical management

The Clinical Management domain is where most marks are lost – often because of time lost in the Data-Gathering phase. Most candidates do the history-taking really well and do it confidently. But the danger is that it becomes a comfort zone they don't want to leave! *Generally speaking* you should be getting into the Clinical Management zone by 6 minutes, and you need to have the competence and confidence to be moving the consultation on without appearing to rush by that time.

Prescriptions and fit notes can potentially form part of the management and completing them well may contribute to your marks. Write them on the forms provided and give them to the patient. If advising investigations and referrals, tell the patient what you intend to do. Information leaflets, diet sheets and so on can be 'sent' or '*collected from the reception desk*'. In time, this rather artificial process may be 'written out' of the exam, but for the time being it remains a CSA exam convention. Suggesting a leaflet should complement good and agreed explanation – it should not be a substitute made in a rush because you are running out of time.

In most cases when prescribing, it is sufficient to tell the patient verbally (and, therefore, the examiner too!) what medication you are prescribing, details of the dosage, how to take it and so on. It is not usually necessary actually to write the script. This too can be 'collected from reception'.

In order to test accurate prescribing, however, some cases require you to write the script there and then. The patient will ask for this to be done, and your script will be assessed for accuracy.

In real-life GP surgeries, of course, EPS (electronic prescriptions) cannot be generated for certain drugs, for example morphine derivatives and tramadol, and this may be reflected in the CSA.

Prescribe correctly and legibly using generic names. By all means use your BNF but avoid spending ages checking formulations and pack sizes, as this will take up valuable consultation time. We are more concerned to see you choosing appropriate drugs and instructing the patient how to take them and good safe practice.

Interpersonal skills (IPS)

Most candidates feel this is an area of strength, indeed most display competence in this domain. As already stated, IPS are assessed from the off in every case, and first impressions count! Be prepared and 'centred' from your review of the patient's records. Temper your greeting.

Listen actively and 'tune in' to the patients wavelength. Respond appropriately to the patient's body language and be conscious of your own. Show concern and interest in symptoms, in how they relate to the patient's world and how they are affected by them. Explore work and what people do, or did, if they are retired, and ask children about school.

Examine professionally, and courteously explain what you are doing and why. Offer chaperoning. At all times, consider the impact of touch and avoid casual use of it.

Reassure and explain where indicated from evidence gathered and reflected on with the patient (scientia), intervene appropriately and show concern for continuity of care and follow-up (caritas).

Ending the consultation

A consultation will often naturally finish early and everything seems to have been accomplished. You can safety-net by asking the patient if all their concerns have been covered and checking their understanding of the agreed plan.

There's no need to pad out the time by throwing in irrelevant health promotion. However, if you seem to have finished in 5 minutes or less, there is a chance that you may have missed something!

LEARNING POINT 27: Re-calling the patient

If a consultation ends before the 10 minutes are up, the patient may leave. If, however, you then suddenly realise you want to cover something else or to correct an aspect of your management, it is absolutely fine within the 10 minutes allowed for the case, to retrieve your patient from the 'waiting room'. Role-players and examiners are under strict instruction to wait outside your door and your marks will not be given until the 10-minute buzzer sounds. This might make a difference to your marks if, for example, you show that you recognise you have recommended an inappropriate drug (allergy?/interaction?).

If the consultation lasts the full 10 minutes, at the closing buzzer/bell the patient will thank you and rise to leave. There is no point in detaining them because you cannot score any more marks after the bell has rung.

LEARNING POINT 28: The 2 minutes between cases

Ctrl + Alt + Delete

Take a deep breath and use the 2-minute break for 'housekeeping'. Clear your mind of the previous case – even if you think you have messed it up, don't waste time agonising about what you should or shouldn't have done! The chances are you did better than you think anyway!

So, 'Control/Alt/Delete'! Regain your composure and move on to look at the records of the next case. Start data-gathering again.

Marking

Examiners refer to a marking schedule for each case, which is a guide to the allocation of marks. These are word-pictures, positive and negative indicators of good and poor performance such as '*Candidate discovers patient's fear that pain is due to heart disease like his father had*' or '*Candidate gathers insufficient data to exclude depression*'. These indicators help the assessor to award-marking grades and they are a framework for marking consistency.

The interpretation of the case-specific marking schedule will have been discussed and agreed as part of the early morning case calibration meeting (see Part 2 for examples and see also the RCGP generic grade descriptors).

For each domain (DG, CM, IPS), examiners will give one of four grades: Clear Pass, Pass, Fail, Clear Fail.

Grades also have descriptors. Here, for example, is one for a marginal pass in the clinical management domain:-

> '*The candidate demonstrates an adequate level of competence, displaying a clinical approach that may not be fluent, but is justifiable and coherent*'.

And here is a descriptor for a marginal fail in the IPS domain:

> '*The patient is treated with sensitivity and respect, but the doctor does not sufficiently facilitate or respond to the patient's contribution.*'

These grades equate to marks as follows – Clear pass = 3, Pass = 2, Fail = 1, Clear Fail = 0. Thus, your performance in each of the three domains (DG, CM, IPS) will be separately rated out of 3. So, for each case in the exam, you will be awarded 0–9 marks.

Rumours circulate about examiners being 'Hawks' or 'Doves', but it is best not to be distracted by such debate and to focus on the patient and the case. For the Harry Potter fans, the Dumbledores and McGelliots co-starring in your appearance at the 'Ministry of Magic' far outnumber the apparent Snapes, and even the Snapes turn out not to be such bad guys!

In essence, think positively and aim for a Clear Pass in all three domains – that is 9 marks in all 13 cases!

Feedback

Examiners are encouraged to give feedback to all candidates and they have to give domain-specific feedback, if they give you failing marks in that domain. They have to do this in the 2 minutes between cases – which can be challenging. It is worth studying the detailed, generic CSA feedback statements available on the RCGP website. These get updated from time to time. Candidates clearly read these, and it has resulted in some tendency towards formulaic consulting – for example, '*Is it OK if I now ask you some specific questions?*' Try to look at these statements and invert them positively (see Chapter 6). This exercise will result in essence in a new personal consultation model 'the CSA model consultation'.

If at first you don't succeed ... You can!

From August 2010, a CSA pass is valid indefinitely. But the number of attempts is now limited to maximum of 4 (if starting GPSTP after August 2010).

Those who succeed in all elements will ultimately be recommended for the CCT. For the small minority who do not succeed, it will be decided if they can have an extension of training to sit the CSA or other components again.

No assessment is perfect, no assessor is perfect, no candidate and no doctor is either, and life events may conspire to impact upon performance through no fault of candidates own. Should you anticipate difficulty or be unfortunate enough not to be successful at your first attempt, please consider the recommendations and advice in Chapter 7 to generate an action plan. To fail to plan is to plan to fail, and there is plenty of support available to help you plan not just to pass but to support you in achieving the excellence we should all be striving for first time. For those who don't pass first time – with the right attitude, approach and educational support, many go on to pass with significantly improved scores.

The intention of the MRCGP is to establish whether, at the time of the individual assessments, you have attained a sufficient level of competence, as measured by the tools available, for you to be 'let loose' as GP on the general public. These include some assessment as to the likelihood of you remaining competent, but current trends, notwithstanding expense to the public and profession, suggest that revalidation will lead in time on to a process of relicensing, which may include AKT and CSA elements – so learn to love the 'CSA model' and aim to carry forward into practice the learning and enjoyment in consulting that a positive approach to it will bring you.

Breaking the consultation up into phases, applying any model is arbitrary and artificial, and it endangers perpetuating a mechanistic approach to consulting. However, the exercise does provide a useful framework for approaching the assessment and consulting in practice. It is important to appreciate that IPS in particular are being continuously assessed from the off – so get off to a good start. You will be at an advantage if performance anxiety doesn't throw you – especially in the first few cases – and if you can keep your head.

Prepare well, feel at home in the 'Euston Square Practice', attend to the recommendations throughout this book, listen to your ethical and interpersonal 'mojo', and visualise yourself as passing. The data will almost gather itself, and you and the patient will reach a clinical management plan seamlessly. 9 marks are there for the taking!

Tips and Hints – On the Day

3.i Reducing Stress on the Day

- Allow enough time to get to Euston, train is best.
- Arrive on time – don't arrive too early or too late.
- Don't forget your I.D.
- Don't forget your examination kit – check the instructions for what to bring.
- If you have a disability, declare this on application.
- If you are sick or acutely stressed, consider deferring.
- Don't take the exam way before you are ready … it's expensive!
- Before your exam, go on a CSA Preparation course – if possible, one which gives a tour of the Exam Centre at Euston so that you know (visually) what to expect.
- Dress professionally, but for comfort.
- Let marshals know if you need to take medication in with you.
- Canteen facilities are limited – but there are snack bars and cafes close by.

During the Exam

- Ignore any observers – they are not there to look at you personally – but at the actor or the case.
- Behave normally and professionally.
- Remember you feel more anxious than you look.
- Don't panic if things go wrong – they probably didn't go as badly as you think!
- Remember housekeeping! Don't carry worries from one case into the next.
- You won't be the only one feeling stressed about a difficult case.
- Ignore the camera.
- Consultations are recorded for the purposes of training examiners and role-players.
- They are not taken to review your performance or grades, and are not available to candidates after the exam.
- They will not be released to others either – for example the deanery.

3.ii Avoid Disqualification

- Before the exam, mobiles, electronic equipment, books and so on must be left in personal lockers provided for each candidate.
- Being found on the exam circuits with notes, textbooks, PDAs, laptops, mobile phones could lead to disqualification.

- Apart from a BNF, no books are allowed.
- You will be asked to sign a confidentiality agreement before sitting the exam.
- Don't remove paperwork, don't take photos of materials.
- Don't talk about cases.
- Read the information about copyright.
- Beware of arousing GMC interest.

3.iii Where Candidates Go Wrong

- Poor time management.
- Poor clinical management plans – unclear or incorrect.
- Management plans are omitted (usually due to lack of time).
- Management plans are not shared with the patient.
- Too narrow a focus – making assumptions too quickly.
- Physical examinations – too much, too little, or simply wrong.
- Getting in a panic.
- Consulting with the examiner, not the patient.
- Not knowing – or appearing not to know – enough general practice.
- Not having had enough exposure – or the wrong kind of exposure – or experience.
- Not knowing the anatomy of the exam and the curriculum.
- Not going on a CSA Preparation course or not having done a consultation skills course.
- Failing to connect with the patient and/or the problem.
- Lacking 'caritas'.

3.iv Maximizing Your Potential

- Integrate your knowledge, skills and attitudes.
- Clinical and communication skills are important – but do not focus entirely on one to the detriment of another.
- Use your skills as a GP to work out what the priorities of the particular consultation are.
- Use your head (knowledge and experience) and use the patient!
- Get the clinical management started by 6 minutes.
- Cue it – for example '*what did you think we might do?*' (while or after examining).
- Guidelines are not rigid protocols.
- Make sure the patient's ICE are taken into account.
- Demonstrate clearly an attempt at shared decision making.
- '*Did you have any thoughts about what we could/should do about this . . .*'

- *'How would you feel, if we … ?*
- *'Could we involve x?'*
- For dilemmas – *'This is a difficult situation. Can you see any way we can work together to find a way forward … ?'*
- Or – *'Is there a possibility for us to work together here to improve things, and at the same time take the opportunity to address your health in general?'*
- It is fine to refer the patient to other health-care professionals – but explain the reason to the patient.
- Explain any PILs you are giving to the patient.

Chapter 4 **Dealing with challenging situations**

You all want to pass the CSA exam. Our best tip is for you to aim to be the best GP possible, and a desirable side effect of this is that you will pass. The question you will ask is how to be the best GP possible?

You should attempt to do regular PR's (not Per Rectal examinations!) but P = Practise and see as many patients as you can; R = Reflect on your cases. This will prepare you for LLL = Life-Long Learning).

You may ask, where is the evidence for 'PR' learning? Perhaps the best illustration of this is in sports. The grandslam champion Roger Federer, won Wimbledon five times, and, therefore, there is no question that he was the best in the world on a grass tennis court. A commentator after another victory in a grandslam final asked how the match had gone and Federer's reply was humble as usual, but he added that there were still areas of his game where he could improve. What we can learn from this is that, even if you're the best GP in the world, it is still worth trying to improve the service you give your patients.

Reflective practice is about reflecting on practice (remember Roger Federer) with reference to clinical and ethical aspects, and showing your trainer that you are doing this on a day-to-day basis. Demonstrating your capacity to build and maintain relationships with patients and colleagues is also the essence of being a good GP – and, among other things, the CSA attempts to assess this capacity.

Everyone can read about ethics; however, application requires examples and experiential learning. We make no apologies, therefore, for a format with more questions than answers.

This chapter is divided into four areas to help you deal with challenges and ethical dilemmas:

1 General principles
2 Areas of application

The CSA Exam: Maximizing your Success, First Edition. Rachel Roberts.

Companion Website: www.wiley.com\go\Roberts\CSAExam

3 Practical Systematic Approach to Ethical Dilemmas (PSA 2 EDs)
4 Case scenarios.

General principles

Think back on last week and consider how many consultations had an ethical element?

One would hope there would be obvious ethical dilemmas; either patient issues, team issues and/or system issues within the NHS (see list under 'Areas of application').

Is there ever a consultation where there is no ethical dimension?

For the purist, every consultation will have some ethical dimension. With even simple presentations of a sore throat, you have to decide to prescribe or not to prescribe antibiotics (perhaps using the Centor criteria for objective assessment), but at the same time you must consider the patient's individual situation (e.g. a patient on immune suppressive drugs) and demands (e.g. '… But doctor, I am going on holiday and cannot have a sore throat').

With the CSA, the 13 cases are likely to be moderate to high challenge (it is an assessment after all), and most failures occur in management rather than data-gathering and interpersonal skills. To increase your chances of success, it is important you grasp the nub of the challenge and the ethical elements to cases, and that you are comfortable dealing with them. In short, candidates who appear to have the experience of doing so, do better, it gives them the 'edge'. This edge only comes with practice – the more patients you see, the more you volunteer to see difficult patients and reflect on these with your trainer, the closer you get to the achieving the 'edge'.

The 13 cases you will see in the CSA are similar to cases you see everyday, and some cases will have more of an ethical dimension than others. Situational Judgement Testing – with which you are all familiar in Foundation programmes – is based on GMC guidance. Think of the CSA in similar terms, that is not as if there are necessarily right or wrong answers, you simply need to make the best decisions in partnership with the patient, and these decisions must be ethically driven – not just being a GP, or a good enough GP, but being a Good GP 13 times in a row.

Why do all GPs go AAR!? AAR – Assessment> Appraisal> Revalidation – this is an ongoing process and, as an ST3 doctor, you will have the triad of assessments: AKT, the CSA and WBA. Having obtained CCT, you will progress to having annual Appraisals followed by 5-yearly Revalidation.

The AAR (assessment, appraisal, revalidation) are only tools to encourage LLL (Life-Long Learning) which subsequently translates to better patient care (Beneficence and Non-maleficence). Furthermore, the ongoing challenge of making the care of our patients the first concern, and balancing/reconciling this with the needs of the practice population and those of the wider society, while being aware of personal views, beliefs and values (Autonomy and Justice).

An analogy which might illustrate medical ethics is a large iceberg floating in water. The tip of the iceberg represents the four basic principles of *autonomy, beneficence, non-maleficence* and *justice;* and below the water, constantly flowing and changing, are the *VALUES* (Toon, 2002; Petrova, 2006) which are inherently involved in our decision making.

LEARNING POINT 29: Upon what values do we base our decisions?
This is not an exhaustive list of underlying VALUES. However, it may help dissect and direct the solving of dilemmas:

- Professional values, for example GMC guidelines/Good medical practice
- Evidence-based medicine, for example NICE and other guidelines
- Legal values – the laws of the country
- Cultural and religious values
- International law
- Moral convictions

Professional values – please read a summary of GMC guidelines. There will be scenarios later illustrating the use of professional values – particularly good medical practice.

Evidence-based medicine – for example, more than a decade ago, a patient suffering with aortic stenosis who was not fit for surgery would have had a very poor prognosis – worse than many cancers – and, therefore, doctors would be discussing palliative care and end-of-life issues. Today, you see the same patient and explain they would do very well with TAVI (transcatheter aortic valve implantation).

Legal values – for example, some countries do not allow termination of pregnancy and this gives women limited choice. Very few countries offer legalised euthanasia and in those circumstances doctors have to be aware if patients want to travel to Swiss or Belgian euthanasia clinics.

Cultural and religious values – for example, be aware that Jehovah's Witnesses may or may not want blood or blood products – but make no assumptions, always ask the patient. (Remember, when you 'assume' – you make an 'ass of U & me')!

International law – for example, we all travel on 'planes, trains and automobiles. If you come across a medical emergency and you are the attending doctor, it is good practice to announce who you are, your speciality, whether you have had any alcoholic beverages or anything else that may affect your judgement, and ask patient's permission if they would like your assistance in the circumstances.

Moral convictions – the attending doctor must always enquire about the patient's perspective and be fully aware of his or her own beliefs and prejudices, and able to offer impartial advice.

LEARNING POINT 30: Go back to your e-portfolio

Look at compliments/SEAs/complaints.

Reflect on them and ask what can be learnt from them ... and how that learning might be tested in a CSA case?

Think about discussions you may ever have had with your indemnity provider and why you had them? What advice did they give you? In doing so, what reference did they make to your 'Duty as a Doctor' and 'Good Medical Practice'?

Areas of application

Broadly speaking in the CSA, as in General Practice, there are three main areas for ethical challenges (just as the three Musketeers, these three areas can be inexorably linked or occasionally separate!).

PATIENT issues – listed chronologically – preconception (e.g. *in vitro* fertilisation, surrogacy, pre-natal screening, etc.), pregnancy (e.g. chorionic villous sampling, termination of pregnancy, demanding elective caesarean, etc.), children (e.g. child protection/safe-guarding issues, consent – Fraser competence (see UPSSIC – Appendix 1), adults [e.g. consent capacity, and being aware when to use the Mental Capacity Act, (see U R x 7 – Appendix 2) versus Mental Health Act , confidentiality, etc.], end-of-life issues (e.g. discussion DNAR – do not attempt resuscitation, organ donation, euthanasia, etc.).

TEAM issues – this could be with your fellow colleagues or other team members, and these can range from poor communication, dishonesty, inappropriate referrals, recurrently starting late, sickness (particularly on Mondays and Fridays), and perhaps the most difficult is whistle-blowing, as illustrated by the 2013 Mid-Staffordshire Hospital crises.

SYSTEM issues – these could be financial and clinical governance issues (e.g. many practices are underpaid by their local health authorities while equally some are overpaid – and how many practices report and return overpayments?), the new dilemmas of referring to NHS or private providers (e.g. if you're a shareholder in the private provider), as a member of the CCG – dealing with conflict of interest with commissioning decisions, rationing of high-value treatments and drugs.

Now that we have briefly discussed the basic principles, the values and the areas where challenging and ethical dilemmas may occur; do you have a systematic way of analysing these problems?

Practical systematic approach to ethical dilemmas (PSA 2 EDs)

In the CSA, any problem is likely to have medical, psychological, social and/or administrative issues. Your task is to discuss with your patient what options are available for management which is acceptable to you, the doctor and also the patient.

Wherever there are options, there is likely to be an ethical construct.

You should find general practice is 'A RIOT' (fun), because there are only five Management options –

A – Ask for advice; *R* – Refer; *I* – Investigate; *O* – Observe; *T* – Treat (*A RIOT*).

However, in reality, you see a common presentation of a sore throat which you, the GP, believe is viral, but the patient is keen to receive antibiotics. There are three common options:

1. You spend time explaining the symptomatic treatment of self-limiting viral illness.
2. In pursuit of patient satisfaction, you give antibiotics – the patient is happy and you are happy as the consultation finishes early.
3. As option 1 above, but you also give a delayed antibiotic prescription.

Let us consider the three management options using the *PSA 2 EDs* – please see the following table where

Y = Yes, generally acceptable
N = Not generally acceptable
? = For discussion/debate
N/A = Not applicable

	Option 1	Option 2	Option 3
	No antibiotic	Give antibiotic	Delay antibiotic
Autonomy	?	y	Y
Beneficience	Y	N	Y
Non-maleficence	Y	N	Y
Justice	N/A	N/A	N/A
VALUES underlying			
Professional GMC	Y	N	Y
Evidence-based medicine	Y	N	Y
Legal values – law	N/A	N/A	N/A
Cultural and religious values	N/A	N/A	N/A
International law	N/A	N/A	N/A
Moral convictions	N/A	?	N/A
Total	4Y, 1?	1Y, 4N, 1?	5Y

As a brief glance at the above table suggests, option 1 and option 3 are more acceptable management plans.

Clearly, in the CSA exam situation, there isn't time to draw this table! However, if during your normal surgeries and weekly tutorial you are able to reflect back on some difficult cases and at times use a 'PSA 2 EDs' – a practical systematic approach to your variable management options – with practice, you can only improve.

LEARNING POINT 31: So, what sort of questions should you be asking yourself?

Every consultation has implicit ethical issues, but you must be aware of, and be prepared to discuss, the explicit issues.

- Is your appointment system too easy or too difficult to access?
- Is your hospital over- or under-treating?

- What is the balance in the decision making in your CCG – patient care versus balancing budget … what are your attitudes, those of colleagues, those of your trainer, partners, salaried, examiners, … how and what might make these change over time … and with reducing resources?

Case scenarios which you could face in general practice

The first few minutes (the data-gathering phase) of each of the scenarios below have been filmed and the video clips are available on our website as an additional learning resource. Our recommendations as to how you might use the clips can be found in the Introduction to Part 2.

N.B. you may wish to view the clips before you read the following text.

Case 1

A 55-year-old unemployed labourer has a flesh wound on his hand. He has been increasingly using heroin and cocaine, is having money problems because he lost his job, and admits to cutting his hand during a recent burglary attempt.

Options

1. Treat the patient for his laceration, drug dependency, depression. Refer to CAB.
2. Same as option 1 plus inform police.
3. Same as option 1 + discuss with colleagues and defence union adviser.

Case 2

John Dyson's only daughter, Gail, a 17 years old, left home last year, after a row, to live with her boyfriend, Darren, 20 years old. Gail's father comes to see you, because he has heard from one of Gail's close friends that Gail is pregnant and Darren has a history of violence. He is worried that Darren may be violent towards Gail. He is hoping you will tell him his daughter's address because she's not answering his calls.

Options

1. Do not give any information to father.
2. Give the father the daughter's contact address.

3 Suggest father contact her friend who can inform his daughter about his concerns.
4 GP to contact patient regarding her father's concerns and offer help such as women's refuge.
5 Same as option 4 + discuss with colleagues and the defence union adviser.

Case 3

The Practice Manager in your surgery asks to talk to you (one of the GPs) confidentially. The Community Nurse of many years standing (15) in the Practice has been behaving erratically.

- It has been noted that she occasionally forgets to visit Patients.
- She, from time to time, arrives late to Clinics with no adequate excuse.
- There have been minor accidents with her car.
- A local Pharmacist has expressed to you in confidence that he is suspicious of drug misuse. She has presented prescriptions on behalf of patients she visits for controlled drugs, and some of these prescriptions have been duplicates issued at her request.

Options

1 Suspend the nurse from duties pending investigations and/or nurse to see her own GP.
2 Let the nurse carry on while investigating and/or nurse to see own GP.
3 Tell the pharmacist to report the nurse.
4 Same as option 1 + discuss with colleagues and defence union adviser.

Case 4

You receive a telephone call from a local pharmacist, who wants to check on one of your scripts. Simon Miller, 26 years old, has presented a prescription signed by you for 300 dihydrocodeine tablets. The pharmacist believes that the number has been altered. You recall prescribing only 30 tablets as analgesics for low back pain.

Options

1 Instruct pharmacist to issue only 30 tablets as per original prescription. Make a note in patient's records about the conversation with the pharmacist.

Arrange to see patient with routine appointment and discuss further management.

2 Ask pharmacist not to issue the prescription at all.
3 Write to patient and take them off your list due to loss of trust in doctor–patient relationship.
4 Same as option 1 + discuss with colleagues and defence union adviser.

Case 5

GP, as patient, requests citalopram because he has been self-medicating for depression. Not suicidal, but possible patient safety concerns at work due to concentration.

Options

1 Prescribe citalopram and convince GP to take time off work; arrange review.
2 Refuse to prescribe citalopram and inform GMC/local health authority.
3 Prescribe citalopram but try to convince GP to inform GMC/health authority.
4 Prescribe citalopram and refer to psychiatry.
5 Option 1 + discuss with colleague and defence union.

Case 6

On a home visit to elderly lady with dementia who has pneumonia, the GP's preference is to admit – but her son and relatives want her to stay home as per her wishes. There is no advanced directive.

Options

1 If GP is convinced the patient wishes to stay home – then treat at home and involve intermediate care team or palliative care team to look after patient.
2 If GP is uncertain, perhaps consider involving 'care of elderly' physician for second opinion.
3 Option 1 or 2 + discuss with colleagues and/or defence union.

In summary – here are three tips to improve your chances of success in the ethical dimension of the CSA:

1 See as many patients as you can (volunteer for difficult patients and home visits).

2 Discuss challenging patients and your video consultations with your trainer regularly.
3 Make time for regular reflection on your e-portfolio. It is most important to document things which have gone well so that you reinforce and anchor your good practice – but you must also be prepared to reflect, change and improve.

Abbreviations

PR	Practice and Reflection
LLL	Life-Long Learning
AAR	Assessment > Appraisal > Revalidation
A RIOT	A – Ask for advice, R – Refer, I – Investigate, O – Observe, T –Treat
PSA 2 EDs	Practical Systematic Approach to Ethical Dilemmas

Appendix 1

UPSSIC
Prof. John Guillebaud (2007) – Fraser Competence assessment – UPSSIC.

You might find it easier to use the acronym in reverse – start off with C – explain to patient the consultation is C-onfidential; explain that, as the GP, it is our priority to make the patient's care our main I-nterest; try to gather information whether the patient is already S-exually active or planning to be, ensure the patient is not likely to S-uffer, such as sexual exploitation or being trafficked; try to encourage the patient to involve someone in P-arental responsibility (could be either parent or older sibling or relative); finally, make sure patient U-nderstands and you as a clinician have to decide whether or not it is justifiable to prescribe.

Appendix 2

UR x 7.

Capacity assessment made really easy *U*sing the magnificent seven *R*s.

First, you ensure patient *Understands* you and exclude any medical disorders which may affect decision-making such as ongoing deafness, depression, delirium and drugs.

Then you can ask the patient – *the 7 Rs.*

*R*etain – can they *retain the information?*
*R*elate – this *relates specifically to the issue you are discussing.*

Recall and Reason – can they *recall the information you give them* and *reason with logic which may not be the same as yours* – or what would be regarded as conventional wisdom but as long as the patient has insight and awareness of the consequences of their decision.

Repeat – can the patient *communicate back to you* the consequences of the decision they have made versus the decision you may be suggesting?

Relative – if a patient is making a decision which is counter to normal wisdom, it is prudent to involve, with the patient's permission, a *relative or close friend* to further discuss this and they may or may not be able to convince the patient to follow your advice.

Reflect – on such a case with *a colleague and/or your defence union.*

References

Guillebaud, J. (2007) "Contraception Today", Informa Healthcare.

"Institute of Medical Ethics". Retrieved 2014, from www.instituteofmedicalethics.org.

Petrova, D.F. (2006) "Values based practice in primary care: easing the tensions between individual values, ethical principles and best evidence" Br J Gen Pract 56: 703–709.

Toon, P. (2002) "Defining & cultivating the virtues" Br J Gen Pract 52: 782–783.

Chapter 5 **Creating and role-playing your own CSA-type case**

Now that we have explored the perspective of you, the candidate, the simulated patient, and the assessment, and discussed how to prepare for and approach potential challenge areas and dilemmas, it is timely to consider a practical exercise to bring all this together, drawing on the rich resource of your day-to-day experience in practice.

This chapter outlines an exercise for training and small-group work that will familiarise you with the basic structure of a CSA case, and enable you to see the exam from all three perspectives. By creating, and then role-playing, CSA-type cases, you will understand how cases are designed and written, how the actors are prepared for their role and how the examiners mark. Then you can practise using these cases in your training and study groups.

The exercise produces three outputs:

1. C – notes for the Candidate – as might appear on the iPad in the CSA.
2. S – notes for the Simulated Patient – role-player briefing notes.
3. A – notes for the Assessor – the marking schedule.

Choose a scenario

Think of the patients you have seen in your surgery in the previous 10 days and the problems or issues they came with. Perhaps a case from your log entries, a recent COT or CBD? Which of those would make a good scenario for a CSA-type case? Remember that it should not be overcomplicated. When this exercise is conducted in groups, our experience is generally that dilemmas and ethical challenge very quickly emerge from even the simplest case; the challenge is to keep it simple.

The CSA Exam: Maximizing your Success, First Edition. Rachel Roberts.

Companion Website: www.wiley.com\go\Roberts\CSAExam

CSA cases will usually contain just the single issue – the 'patient's' opening statement usually reflects accurately what the case is about, but there is often additional clinical and ethical meat on the bones.

You – or one of your fellow trainees – will have to role-play this 'patient'. Preferably, the gender should be the same, because it helps credibility when it comes to the role-play. In the CSA, the role-player will 'look the part' – that is the 'patient's' gender, age, ethnicity, BMI and other physical characteristics will reflect what is written in the patient records on the candidate's iPad. However, it is worth pointing out that in the pre-exam briefing, candidates are told that unforeseen circumstances can arise on the day of the exam itself – an actor may be taken ill, for example, and need to be replaced by one who does not 'look the part'. In those circumstances, candidates are advised to go by what is written on the patient records and not by the shape or age of the role-player in front of them. So even the gender is not essential as long as the 'candidate' consults with the 'patient' as outlined in the patient records!

Notes for the candidate

At this point sketch up the 'Notes for the Candidate' – the kind of information you should be reading from the iPad in the all important 2-minute Housekeeping start-up phase to your CSA consultations. Typically, this will comprise

- Name
- Age, Gender
- Past Medical History
- Drug History and Allergies
- Family and Social History
- Last Consultation
- Relevant Results/Correspondence

(see the Case paperwork in Part 2 for guidance).

Briefing the role-player

Once you have chosen your scenario for the case, you will need to spend 10–15 minutes filling out the background details for the role-player who is going to portray the 'patient'. Initially, these might be based on the real patient you had in your surgery recently who has inspired you to develop this case. What are the symptoms/problems which brought the patient to come to see you, that is what is his/her agenda? What, therefore, is an appropriate opening statement, and with what tone of voice and body language/ demeanour will that be delivered?

Whoever is to role-play the case will need to know simple personal details (e.g. age) and details about family and work, where the problems might be having an impact. What are the patient's social, psycho-social background, ideas, concerns and expectations (remember SPICE!). It's in the SPICE that you may find the source of problems, as well as clues to the approach to management solutions for the patient. All CSA actors will be briefed to give answers about these as long as the candidate prompts them appropriately and sensitively.

You may anticipate other questions which a candidate might pose, given this scenario, so your role-player needs to be briefed how to answer. Similarly, are there questions which the patient in this situation would ask the doctor?

Does your case entail physical examination? If so, are you as a case-writer expecting this examination to be done within the 10 minutes, or is your 'candidate' going to need a handout with findings or results?

Are there other resources you will need to make this case run realistically, examination equipment/peak flow charts/growth charts/letters and so on.

Outline details for the role-player briefing notes

- Symptoms/problem
- Opening statement
- Demeanour and tone
- Background details – personal/family/work
- Answers to anticipated questions from doctor
- Questions to ask the doctor
- Physical examination handouts (if appropriate)
- Patient record sheet (to be given to the 'candidate')

Marking schedule

Now that you have briefed your 'patient', you need to focus on the 'candidate', and start to wear your 'examiner's cap'. As you will by now be aware, CSA cases are marked in three separate domains – data-gathering, clinical management and interpersonal skills (see Chapter 3). For each of these domains, you will need to brainstorm what you expect the 'candidate' to do in response to the 'patient's' symptoms/problems. It may be useful to skip ahead to Part 2 to see some examples of this in the case 'palette'.

If you have one available, write notes up on a flipchart so that you can refer to them after the case has run. Spend about 10–15 minutes on this part of the exercise.

Data-gathering – what questions (open and closed) does the doctor have to ask in order to take an adequate history, given the opening statement and the 'patient's' agenda? Is physical or mental examination needed?

Clinical management – what is appropriate in this situation? Think about evidence-based practice and how the doctor may deal with any dilemma or ethical issues, and what your criteria for competence are.

Interpersonal skills – these tend to be generic, so try to be as specific as possible to the case scenario.

Resources on the RCGP CSA website, you may find useful to reflect on, as part of this exercise are as follows:

- Generic indicators for targeted assessment domains
- Analysis of passing and failing candidates.

The role-play

So now all you need is a willing (?) volunteer to play the 'candidate'!

Ideally, it should be a member of your study group who wasn't involved in the above preparation – or, even better, a trainee you don't know well! Firstly, it is more beneficial for the 'candidate' to approach the case as in the CSA itself. (S)he has just a couple of minutes to read and reflect on the 'patient-records' you give them before starting the consultation.

Secondly, it is useful for you, the case-writer, to review your marking schedule (and possibly also the way the role-player was briefed) in the light of what actually happened when the case ran. Did the 'candidate' consult in the way you had expected? If not, which of you (case-writer or consulter) can learn from this?

Watching others consult is such a valuable exercise, and you should have no qualms about 'stealing unashamedly' for yourself good techniques or good phrases which others use. At the same time, however, remember Pendleton rules when you give feedback to each other. Emphasise the positives – but be constructively critical about aspects which could be done better.

We have produced a feedback sheet template to assist this exercise (see Appendix to this chapter). In giving feedback, you may also find it useful to make reference to the next chapter which is our re-rendering of the CSA Examiners' feedback statements

Conclusion

A few final points:

- Don't overcomplicate the medical scenario you choose. Most CSA cases are straightforward – dilemmas or challenges, if present, will be overt.
- The simulated 'patient' must remember to play the 'uninformed patient' who should question jargon or medical terminology which a lay person would not understand.
- Role-playing is different from acting. It is important to play the 'patient' as naturally and realistically as possible. Try to get inside the head of this 'patient' and understand their SPICE.
- Don't overact the 'patient' or the GP – even if you have an audience! Whichever chair you are sitting in, be yourself and act naturally – and this applies in the CSA itself too.

Creating and writing a CSA-type case format of the exercise

Choose a scenario – something you encountered in the previous 10 days? (5 minutes)

Work on the role-player briefing (10–15 minutes): *Need a 'volunteer' to role-play the 'patient' later*

Work on the marking schedule (10–15 minutes): *Present this on a flipchart sheet if possible*

Role-play the case: Need volunteer 'candidate' (it's good practice!)

- Act out the case (10 minutes)
- Feedback to the 'candidate'
- Presentation and review of marking schedule
- General discussion and Learning points (10–15 minutes)

In our experience, this 'quick and dirty' exercise is a really valuable – but simple – training tool for you to use in small study groups. We hope you find it useful. Cases on good CSA preparation courses using simulated patients are a quantum leap higher in terms of challenge, not so much because of content, but because of the setting and execution by trained role-players.

In the CSA, the development of individual cases is a sophisticated and painstaking process and will take 18 months or so between the initial draft and going 'live' on the exam circuit. Cases have to be trialled with role-players first and then piloted later with ST3s playing the 'candidate'.

Even after all that time, candidates will still ask unexpected questions for which the actor has not been briefed. In such circumstances, the role-players are trained to give a neutral response – for example 'I don't know'. Sometimes, if they are asked something unexpectedly which the 'patient' would definitely know, but for which they haven't been briefed, then they will 'ad lib', as the CSA actors are trained to do, and give a natural, realistic answer – as long as that answer could not possibly mislead the candidate. This will normally be drawn from their own lives.

In this exercise, it is likely that your role-player will have to ad lib liberally which adds to the fun and should be encouraged – (s)he has only had 10–15 minutes or so to prepare, after all!

Appendix to Chapter 5 – A sample case feedback sheet

Case details		
Domain	Done well	Could be done differently
Data gathering		
Clinical management		
Interpersonal skills		
Global features/comments		
Learning action points Revision tips		

Chapter 6 **Maximizing your potential with feedback from examiners**

All candidates get feedback on their performance in the CSA. This is intended to be formative, but, rather uncomfortably, does not follow the 'Pendleton rules' and is generically couched in the negative in the form of the CSA Candidate Feedback Statements. Recently, the way feedback is given has been reviewed and enhanced within the e-portfolio to improve its formative benefit. It remains the case that examiners only *have* to give feedback if they give a failing mark. The intention of feedback as always is to help reflection on possible areas for improvement, but it is also in a sense true to say that the examiners have to 'justify' giving failing marks by giving this feedback. In future, it is intended that all candidates will receive feedback.

In preparing for the exam, it may pay, therefore, to aim to make it challenging for the examiners to give you negative feedback. It follows that it may be helpful for you, 'to get inside the examiner's head' and turn these statements round, using them as *positive* formative aims, rather than waiting to get them given to you negatively!

We would encourage you to adopt this approach – for example in the small group work exercise outlined in the previous chapter and perhaps with your trainer, using joint surgeries to simulate the CSA. You and your trainer, for example, could take turns role-playing the examiner/candidate conducting a CSA style COT using the feedback sheets (Appendix to Chapter 5) with an eye on the global and domain-specific suggestions in this chapter.

Maximize Your Potential: Use Your Trainer for Feedback in Preparing for the CSA – A Suggested Model for Your Joint Surgeries

The trainer Dr X leaves the consulting room closing the door. The registrar Dr Y reads the notes of the next case 'Housekeeping'.

The CSA Exam: Maximizing your Success, First Edition. Rachel Roberts.

Companion Website: www.wiley.com\go\Roberts\CSAExam

Meanwhile in the waiting room, Dr Y prepares the patient Mrs Z.
'Hello Mrs Z, I am Dr X. Thank you for agreeing to see Dr Y today. Dr Y is preparing for professional exams and I will be observing this (10-minute) consultation. Would you be happy to be involved in a brief feedback discussion at the end of the consultation? (Is that OK? Any questions?) ... please knock and enter'
Registrar starts clock/counter on knock ... ? buzzer at 10 minutes!? Consultation concludes.
Trainer observes and completes CSA COT followed by a facilitated discussion with the patient if appropriate and further feedback. These COTs can later be elaborated on as WBA COTs.

Even if you do well and pass, all candidates get some feedback if the feedback statements are selected by two or more examiners – but generally, it's feedback you don't really want or would rather have had before!

Formative feedback is given in relation to 16 areas of performance (see below). Not all of these are tested in every consultation, although they will be tested across the assessment as a whole. Examiners mark each case and then indicate any areas in which they felt your performance could be better. Any area of performance identified as one for potential improvement by two or more examiners will be flagged. Please note that the feedback you receive is NOT an indication of your marks. High performers may still get some feedback.

Below you will find statements covering the CSA global and individual domains with suggestions as to how to *maximize your potential* based on those feedback statements.

Many of the statements overlap slightly, and being good in one area means you are more likely to be good in another. However, it may also seem that some of the statements are at odds with one another. For example, you may find that exploring the patient's concerns takes time which in turn might lead to you not being able to complete the consultation in the time allowed. It is important to remember that the CSA is a test of your ability *to integrate and apply* your clinical skills to the specific scenario, so that, in order to do well, you need to be able to manage the tensions between different aspects of good consulting – 'all the skills, all the time'.

(Not) The CSA candidate feedback statements

Global-structure, 'nub', time

1. Aim for an organised/structured consultation

Your consultation follows a logical structure. Your history-taking is a joined-up line of questioning and follows a clearly reasoned way of thinking.

You appear organised, with elements (e.g. health promotion) included, if appropriate.

This gives the impression that you are a doctor whose line of diagnostic thinking and clinical management will address important clinical issues, and that you are systematic.

Practical Suggestions to Help Maximize Your Global Potential

Practising with one of the published consultation models (such as Neighbour, Pendleton or Cambridge-Calgary). Analysing some of your video consultations helps you develop a more fluent approach. Ask a colleague or your trainer to critique your consulting. When taking a history, you should initially listen to the patient and ask open questions to explore the presenting features, before focusing on the specific detail with closed questions, when and if appropriate. It is sometimes helpful to signal to the patient that you are about to do this by saying or signalling something like 'Would it be Ok if I ask you some specific questions now?' But this phrase lifted straight from feedback is getting very hackneyed. Use your own conversational words to say something like – '*I just need to clarify a few things*'.

Explain to the patient what you are doing and why. This is good for patient care and will also demonstrate to examiners that you have a clear and systematic approach. Explaining to the patient exactly what further tests (e.g. blood tests, if appropriate to the case) are going to be necessary for further management, also helps the examiners know what you are planning to do and why, and agreeing the plan with the patient is key.

Summarising aspects of the information you have collected also demonstrates to examiners that you are collating and processing data, and is useful in checking with the patient that you have understood. A phrase such as – 'So, just to summarise' – at certain points may give an impression of reflecting and formulating information received or actions agreed.

2. Recognise the issues or priorities in the consultation (e.g. the patient's problem, ethical dilemma)

Demonstrate that you are able to identify the patient's problem/agenda or the possible challenges in the consultation and appropriate priorities from the doctor's perspective. Pick up on the aspects to the case that need to be covered, in addition to the superficial clinical presentation. For example, if a patient presents with a possible sexually transmitted infection, i.e. an STI, the consultation should include sensitive enquiry about the likelihood of this (addressing the patient's worries) AND a section on contact-tracing, and whether a partner (addressing the wider ethical dilemma).

Practical Suggestions to Help Maximize Your Potential to Recognise Priorities

Patients don't always tell you straight away what is worrying them, and may have to be asked. Sometimes, the way they look, what they say, or how they say it gives you clues to an underlying worry. There may be a situation that has an ethical dimension to it that the patient may not have considered, but that you, as a professional, are expected to show awareness of, and respond to – for example an issue of confidentiality.

- *Use your e-portfolio to log and reflect on challenging cases.*
- *See lots of cases – get experience.*

Being alert to verbal and non-verbal cues and analysing your consultations either on video or in shared surgeries might help you with this. Look closely at your ability to encourage the patient to share his/her thoughts and expectations. Ask an experienced colleague what they thought the issues and priorities in the consultation were, and discuss how these compare with your opinion. Think about the implications of the presentations you see in your own surgeries, and how they might present in the CSA.
Hidden agendas are NOT common in practice and, despite popular belief, are not a feature of CSA cases. Plenty of consulting experience, case discussion, random case analysis and video work with your trainer will help you cultivate an holistic approach that will help you in the CSA where agendas are far more overt.

3. Use time available well and effectively (in general, aim to get on to the Clinical Management by 6 minutes at the latest)
Housekeeping: read the patient notes on your iPad before the first case. Move on from last case immediately and use the 2 minutes between cases to read the notes and any material for the next case.

Listen actively to the opening statement and observe the patient's tone and demeanour.

Give time, and take time, as appropriate.

Practical Suggestions to Help Maximize Your Potential to Manage Time Effectively

Read the patient notes before consulting each patient – check recent entries, medication, allergies, correspondence. This is a great and time-saving habit instilled by CSA practice that will serve you well in your whole career.

Seeing patients in 10-minute appointments in your own surgeries, and trying to ensure that you remain focused on the problem presented will help. Try to observe doctors who consult effectively and efficiently, and learn how to modify your own approach.

A common reason for running out of time in CSA cases is due to candidates taking too long to take a history, and then having to rush the second half of the consultation – clinical management, explanations and follow-up arrangements. Pace yourself and work out how long you should be taking for the different parts of the consultation.

Gathering information requires you to be appropriately selective in the questions you ask, the tests you request and the examinations you choose to undertake. You may feel that it would be better to be 'on the safe side' by ordering a battery of tests but, while perhaps understandable, this can make you appear indiscriminate. Likewise, history taking and examination is not expected to be all-inclusive and should be tailored to the circumstances and include psycho-social factors where relevant. This will help you greatly in your future clinical practice as well as in the CSA.

Data-gathering, use all the information available, examine well

4. Identify abnormal findings and results, recognise their implications. Read the notes/look at the material/findings/letters/pictures ...

Demonstrate an ability to identify/recognise significant findings in the history, examination or data interpretation from results. Act upon them appropriately, showing you recognise their significance. Issues identified may need to be prioritised clearly.

Practical Suggestions to Help Maximize Your Potential in Data-gathering: Abnormal Findings and Results

This is a clinical rather than interpersonal skill and requires you to make sure that you can correctly interpret the significance of test results or the findings of physical and mental state examinations. The abnormal findings will nearly always relate to common or important conditions, and you should bear in mind that common conditions are more likely than uncommon ones in real life, as well as in the CSA. This should be reflected in the differential diagnosis you make, and in how you explain your differential diagnosis to the patient.

- *Common things occur commonly, but rare things do happen in exams and elsewhere.*

- *Help with day-to-day results and correspondence processing in the practice – 'every little helps' you learn as well as helping the patients and the business.*

When you prepare for the CSA, pay close attention to your ability to assess and manage risk by picking up on abnormal findings and dealing with them safely – that is demonstrate an ability to risk stratify. Discuss your management with colleagues, asking them to comment particularly on your risk management and safety-netting. Also, take an active part in significant event reviews, look back on these, especially if relating to clinical errors and see what you can learn.

- *Use and log your out of hours and extended hours visiting and telephone experience sessions, think about how you safety-net differently in different situations.*
- *Log SEAs and complaints, read the indemnity magazines – construct some practice CSA cases based on these.*

5. Undertake physical examination competently and use instruments proficiently

Hone your physical examination skills. You should be able to demonstrate the appropriate and fluent use of instruments, in a way that does not distress patients, with their full understanding of what you are doing and their consent. Look comfortable and practise competent examining, as if you have done it lots of times.

Be professional and courteous.

Practical Suggestions to Help Maximize Your Potential In data-gathering: Physical Examination

Improving these skills is a matter of practice, and it pays to spend time developing a systematic method that you can repeat over and over again. Before doing so, take advice and make sure that your technique is correct; otherwise you will simply be reinforcing bad habits. Once correct techniques are practised and become fluent, your approach will appear competent and confident to the examiner.

You should always explain what you are proposing to do in an examination to the patient, and why you are doing it. In the case of intimate examinations (they can be indicated in the CSA), you should make sure you have gained informed consent and offered a chaperone.

- COTs will help.
- Joint surgeries will help.
- CSA practice in small groups will help.

Useful websites with helpful clips http://www.pennine-gp-training.co.uk/physical-examination-videos-for-the-csa.htm or http://www.e-lfh.org.uk/home. You will need to get a login for this NHS/RCGP endorsed site and search for 'physical examinations'.

Clinical management, diagnosis, manage uncertainty, risk and safety-netting, be up-to-date, resources, health promotion

6. Make the correct working diagnosis, identify an appropriate range of differential possibilities

Make the appropriate diagnosis. You should consider common conditions in the differential diagnosis.

Practical Suggestions to Help Maximize Your Potential in Clinical Management: Diagnosis and Diagnostic Possibilities

This statement is linked with statement 4:

Recognise abnormal information, either in the history, the examination, or data provided in the case notes.

Making a diagnosis means committing yourself on the basis of the information you have that is available to you. Make sure that your knowledge base is adequate (do some AKT papers in the run-up to the CSA – for example on passmedicine.com), and think carefully about all the information that is presented to you in the case. Then ensure that when you have made a diagnosis in consultation, you state this clearly and explain it to the patient, using language that is understandable to them (see 16). If your summary is too vague, the examiner may not be sure that you have made a diagnosis at all. If you have a differential diagnosis list, explain this to the patient too, remembering that common things occur commonly, and are (usually) more likely! It is not always necessary to make a single diagnosis; you can still do well, provided you explain what you are thinking and why. To say you unsure is OK as long as you explain to the patient how you plan to proceed or to find out the answer to a question they might have asked, and as long as your plan can be understood by the examiner and judged to be safe.

7. Develop a management plan (including prescribing and referral) reflecting knowledge of current best practice

Develop a management plan with the patient and show that your clinical management skills are in line with current UK best practice.

Practical Suggestions to Help Maximize Your Potential in clinical Management: Apply Knowledge of Current Best Practice

Your management plans and follow-up arrangements should reflect the natural history of the condition, and be appropriate to the level of risk. They should be coherent and feasible. You should be aware of up-to-date national guidelines such as those published by NICE (National Institute of Clinical Excellence) and SIGN (Scottish Intercollegiate Guidelines Network), and you should demonstrate you have an evidence-based approach.

Possible risks and benefits of different approaches (including prescribing) need to be clearly identified and discussed. Your knowledge base is also important in this area. Use the concept of PUNs (Patients' Unmet Needs) and DENs (Doctors' Educational Needs) to improve this selectively, and discussing the management of cases you have seen with an experienced doctor will help you in these areas. Your understanding of decisions for referral should also mirror current guidelines and UK best practice.

8. Show appropriate use of resources, including aspects of budgetary governance

Some cases may include an aspect that requires you to demonstrate your role as a 'gate-keeper' of NHS resources. This includes aspects of requests for 'fit notes', surgical procedures, newly developed medications, use of appropriate referral pathways and referrals for second opinions. All of these are the 'bread and butter' of general practice.

Practical Suggestions to Help Maximize Your Potential in Clinical Management: Resources and Budgetary Governance

Discuss this issue with an experienced general practitioner, such as your trainer or one of the partners in the practice. Get to know your local medicines management team or prescribing advisors, they are fonts of useful information. Think about the different types of NHS resources for which GPs are 'gate-keepers', and how reference to them could come up in routine consultations. Get involved in referral audits. Look through your video consultations to identify times when appropriate use of resources has come up – you will find it comes up in nearly every consultation in one way or another. This does not mean that you refuse access to services, new medications or 'fit notes', but that you show your awareness of the issues and responsible use of resources.

Tip: Review GMC guidance. Revise ethics. Balance 'making the best care of the patient being your first concern' with your duty to your practice population, the local community and society as a whole. Practise sharing this with patients and negotiating a way forward. Create an opportunity for partnership-working rather than confrontation.

Think broadly about resources – time, money, drugs, referrals are obvious … information, knowledge, power – 'The Drug Doctor' less obvious. Don't forget that you and your relationships with your patients and other professionals are vital resources too. How far do you share resources, and where are your boundaries? How and when are you flexible with them and why?

9. Make adequate arrangements for follow-up and safety-netting

Practical Suggestions to Help Maximize Your Potential in Clinical Management: Safety-netting

It is easy for consultations to be seen as isolated incidents, rather than a continuum in the course of an illness. Make arrangements for follow-up which demonstrate your commitment to the continuity of care of patients and your concern for their welfare and safety. It also shows that you are prepared to take responsibility for managing the ongoing presentation of the condition until the problem has been resolved in some way.

Safety-netting (coined by Neighbour in the context of the consultation) is a term that describes the explanations you should be giving to each patient about what to expect, including a timescale if appropriate, and about what to do if symptoms get worse or develop in some way that is unexpected. If there is uncertainty about the diagnosis, this should be communicated to the patient so they are empowered to re-consult if necessary. You should include a description of where and how to get help, at any time of day or night, if this seems appropriate for the case being presented, as well as arrangements for follow-up.

10. Demonstrate an awareness of the management of risk, make the patient aware of the relative risks of different options

Manage risk appropriately, identify the potential risks and integrate your risk assessment into the consultation in a useful way which is acceptable to the patient.

Practical Suggestions to Help Maximize Your Potential in Clinical Management: Management of Risk

In order to manage risk appropriately, you should make the patient aware of the relative risks of different approaches. Managing risk and living with uncertainty are key skills in general practice. Your knowledge base is important here, as is your ability to integrate that knowledge with the specific information you have gained about the patient. Listening to how more experienced practitioners explain common risks might be helpful (e.g. the risks of taking Hormone Replacement Therapy). Then practise doing the same in your own words which will help you develop this skill. You don't want to be doing this for the first time in the CSA – an unpractised candidate is very obvious to examiners. Role-play with teachers and fellow trainees would give you a start.

Familiarise your self with biopsychosocial assessment for depression and evaluation of suicidality; be familiar with local safeguarding procedures for children and adults.

11. Attempt to promote good health at opportune times in the consultation

Practical Suggestions to Help Maximize Your Potential in Clinical Management: Opportunistic Health Promotion

Health promotion requires doctors to demonstrate an awareness of health (rather than just illness), and to be proactive in maintaining the patient's health. Try to be aware of health promotion issues and apply these appropriately. The key to doing this successfully is to identify the patient's health beliefs and work with them towards a plan for maintaining good health. The use of computer-generated prompts can sometimes be helpful in order to keep this issue on your agenda during a consultation, but you won't have this benefit in the CSA. You will need to keep health promotion in mind as part of the tasks of the consultation.

The doctor's agenda, for example gathering data for health promotion, is important, but the challenge is to achieve an appropriate balance with the patient's agenda. It is also important that attempts at health promotion are done in an opportune way so that they complement the patient's agenda rather than trying to supersede it. One of the keys to doing this successfully is in the feedback statement '.... *at opportune times in the consultation*'. Just firing off a list of health promotion questions out of context is unlikely to be welcome to the patient and so is unlikely to be effective. It also wastes your consultation time and doesn't score extra marks! Please remember that giving a PIL without explanation to the patient will not gain you any credit. Examiners cannot mark leaflets!

Conversely asking your practice nurse colleagues involved in chronic disease management/doctors in the practice which their favourite leaflets are, printing them off and familiarising yourself with management and treatment options, and the patient-friendly language such advice is usually rendered in on reputable websites can help put a sheen on your clinical management (see statement 12).

Interpersonal skills, rapport, active listening, psycho-social, sharing plans, choosing words well

12. Develop rapport and show awareness of the patient's agenda, health beliefs and preferences

Develop rapport and a good professional relationship with the patient. Demonstrate awareness of the patient's feelings during your history taking and examination. Gather data sensitively. Practise taking a sexual history for example. Identify the patient's agenda, health beliefs and preferences, and apply information to guide the rest of the consultation.

Practical Suggestions to Help Maximize Your Potential in Interpersonal Skills: Patient-centredness

Demonstrating interest in, and warmth towards, the patient and seeking consent for any clinical examination is important. How you develop a rapport depends on factors relating not only to the patient and their situation but also to your personal style preferences. Making eye contact, smiling and welcoming patients into the consultation helps put patients at ease. (However, bouncing out of the chair to shake every patient firmly by the hand may be inappropriate and occasionally culturally offensive.)

Identifying when you achieve rapport with a patient, and working out how you did so can be helpful. Then you can build on your strengths rather than copy how others do it. It is often just a matter of showing a true interest in the patient and their problems by non-verbal as well as verbal communication.

Be kind and appropriately curious and enquiring. Your posture and body language is important.

By 'health beliefs' we mean the reasons underlying the patient's thinking about his/her presentation in the case. It does not need to be investigated exhaustively, but the patient's perspective should be sought.

This skill lies at the heart of patient-centred consulting and a number of educational resources will help you to understand the concept. Consider different consultation models and how you relate to different patients. Being curious about the patient, and trying to understand their perspective will help you to identify their views. This is most effective if integrated into the consultation, and you are more likely to find out about the patient's concerns if you tailor your questions and their timing to each individual.

You could prepare by allowing doctors who are skilled in this approach to assess your performance by, for example, rating you on the COT (consultation observation tool) and providing formative feedback. Build on this by working in small groups and/or video work with your trainer.

Look at your PSQs with your trainer you may be surprised to find areas in which your performance against peers is rated differently – discuss and reflect with your trainer on areas where you could improve or do things differently.

13. Use active-listening skills and respond to cues. Avoid a formulaic approach (slavishly following a model and/or being unresponsive to the patient), be fluent and be responsive

Look out for verbal or non-verbal cues in the consultation to increase your understanding of the patient's situation. Listen actively and avoid repeating questions, but do reflect back and summarise.

Practical Suggestions to Help Maximize Your Potential in Interpersonal Skills: Active Listening and Response to Cues

Active listening includes asking questions at the appropriate time, in a logical sequence in response to the patient's last contribution. It is demonstrated by the good use of verbal and non-verbal cues. Good active listening includes allowing the patient to say what they want to tell you, and sometimes helping them by clarifying and summarising what they have already said (which shows you were listening and have understood them). Video work can be especially helpful to develop these skills.

Recognising cues, both verbal and non-verbal, is a key component of patient-centred clinical method. Cues can include gestures, pauses in speech and facial expressions, as well as clues in the patient's account that indicate he/she has additional issues to tell you. The information gained from acting on patient cues is likely to increase patient satisfaction.

By 'formulaic' consulting, we mean that the doctor appears to be rigidly applying a fixed consulting 'model' to the consultation, which does not take into account the patient's agenda or response. The doctor may repeat questions, ask questions at inappropriate times in the consultation and use unnatural pre-prepared phrases.

Some of these phrases seem to come from CSA courses or CSA guides, as suggestions about how to show empathy or to elicit and manage a patient's concerns or lifted straight out of these feedback statements. Use your own words – be authentic.

To the examiner, especially if it is asked repeatedly during the consultation and then little or no notice is taken of the answer, it appears that such questions are being asked as part of a 'formula' that candidates have learnt to pass the CSA. Such an approach is an inevitable consequence of habituation to a test, and it may just about help you to display mechanical competence. Conversely cultivating a personal approach by all means borrowing and adapting such phrases is likely to come across as more authentic and impressive because ultimately General Practice is about you finding and enjoying a consulting style of your own.

Develop your own 'script' if you want to impress the examiners. Those suggested in the feedback are suggestions not a formula: note they are prefaced with 'something like' – for example 'Would it be Ok if I ask you some specific questions now?' – but you should find your own way of saying things.

This is an area that is sometimes difficult to develop without the help of more experienced doctors. Watching yourself on video, and asking your trainer to review videos with you, is a useful way of seeing yourself as others might observe you. It might also be helpful to gather information about what your patients feel about this aspect of your work before and after you have tried to improve these skills.

14. Identify and use appropriate psychological and/or social information to place the problem in context

Obtain and use existing information about the patient's background in such a way as to increase your understanding of how the problem might affect the patient's everyday life – rather than just their health. The common elements of this 'background' are the patient's psychological state and the influences of their social network, occupation and culture. Ask about work and what work involves doing and how the problem affects what they do.

The best candidates understand the impact the particular problem is having on the patient.

Practical Suggestions to Help Maximize Your Potential in Interpersonal Skills: SPICE

Understanding and appreciating the social and psychological aspects of a patient's problem are key to practising patient-centred medicine. Using a consultation model and reviewing your consultations either alone or with your trainer, paying special attention to this aspect, will help it to become second nature. Similarly, asking yourself a few questions after each consultation will soon enable you to identify whether this is something that you do routinely. Such questions might be: How is the problem affecting the patient? What changes have they had to make to their life because of this problem? Who else is affected by the problem? In addition, ask yourself whether you have any blind spots. For instance, do you ask what the patient's job involves rather than just what their job title is? Are there issues of diversity in the case? People differ in their life experiences. Factors such as social class, ethnicity, age, gender and sexuality play an important part in presentation of illness.

15. Develop a shared management plan, demonstrating an ability to work in partnership with the patient

Demonstrate the development of a shared management plan. Discuss the pros and cons of options, taking account of the patient's views, to aid the development of shared understanding.

Practical Suggestions to Help Maximize Your Potential in Interpersonal Skills: Sharing Your Management Plan

This may be improved by responding appropriately to the patient's agenda and by attempting to involve patients in making decisions regarding their problem. Clarifying the respective roles may involve reaching agreement with the patient as to what will happen next, who does what and when, and the conditions (i.e. the timescale and circumstances) for follow-up. There should be a shared understanding before the patient leaves, and this can be confirmed by asking the patient to summarise what they have understood – [But be careful – this can appear formulaic if done inappropriately!]

How you do this is a matter of finding out what works best for you and taking a lead from the patient. Using standard questions such as 'What will you tell your partner when you get home?' rarely works well, as it is not a common way to talk and sounds artificial (see above). On the other hand, it might be just the right question to ask if you have identified that the patient's partner has a particular concern about their health. Patient-centred doctors are responsive to patient preferences, including when they don't want to share decision making 'You're the doctor, doctor – you tell me', and they work to develop common ground and a shared understanding. There are many educational resources (books, DVDs of consulting skills, etc.) that will help you to achieve this.

16. Use language and/or explanations that are relevant and understandable to the patient

Practical Suggestions to Help Maximize Your Potential in Interpersonal Skills: Language and Explanations

In developing this skill, it is important to avoid the use of jargon to establish the patient's level of understanding of medical and health matters and to tailor your explanation to these. Whether or not your explanation has been understood can be checked through non-verbal communication but also (and more explicitly) by asking the patient to summarise. Explanations are often most effective when you affirm a patient's health beliefs e.g. 'Like you, I think this pain might be due to a trapped nerve ... ' Similarly using the same language as the patient aids understanding and helps to make the patient aware that you have listened to what they have been saying (i.e. echoing/mirroring). It also avoids formulaic consulting and comes across as more conversational and natural. Avoid, or at least, be careful with medical jargon, and check for understanding. If you have difficulty explaining an issue in lay terms, try printing off a patient information leaflet from a reputable website (which will have been written in patient-friendly terms) and memorise the explanations there.

It is also germane to consider how you might communicate with patients with a specific disability such as one of sight, hearing, speech or learning. How might your ability be tested in the CSA? How would you adapt your consultation skills accordingly? Think what language or communication skills might you use and why.

To conclude we hope this comprehensive, re-rendered inversion of the feedback statements helps you in your preparation for the exam, and also to get inside the heads of the examiners and really make them struggle to find any feedback whatsoever to give in that precious 2 minutes in the exam corridor while you are confidently reading the notes of the next case.

Chapter 7 **Strategies for candidate concerns with the CSA**

This chapter aims to help you if you have difficulties or specific concerns regarding your likelihood of passing the CSA. It is designed to help those who feel they have reason to anticipate difficulty, as well as those who find themselves re-sitting the CSA exam. The degree of difficulty can be wide ranging. It may be very mild, so that your scores in preparation are lower than those predicted by your trainers, but still well within the passing range. Or it may be more challenging, with either multiple exam difficulties such as CSA and AKT, or repeated exam re-sits.

LEARNING POINT 32: First steps in addressing candidate concerns

- Identify potential barriers to success
- Develop self awareness
- Enlist appropriate help
- Develop appropriate strategies
- Be aware of available resources.

Anticipating difficulty

In terms of anticipating difficulty before it arises, it is important to differentiate whether you have satisfactory or even good ability to pass the CSA, but simply lack confidence. Other possibilities are that there are issues to resolve in order to allow your success, and that your very sensible strategy is that you would like to address these before your first and hopefully only CSA sitting.

The CSA Exam: Maximizing your Success, First Edition. Rachel Roberts.

Companion Website: www.wiley.com\go\Roberts\CSAExam

In the first instance, we would signpost you to the first chapter in this book, '*Maximizing Potential in the CSA*' regarding full preparation, both psychologically and educationally for maximum performance on the day. Research has shown that self-assessment of ability varies in accuracy depending on a range of factors, from personality to overall ability compared to your peer group. Some people's personalities have a tendency to lack of confidence despite good ability, while others overestimate their ability.

Here it may be worth you trying to remember how your past estimates regarding your ability correlated with that of your trainers', examiners' or assessors' opinions. This may give you a clue to the likely accuracy of your predictions regarding issues to overcome.

Increased insight as to your ability educationally is thought to parallel the increasing development of skills as you progress. Wherever you find yourself in a scale of performance when consulting, please remember it is simply a part of a progression. This means that if you are on the correct path, and progressing at a suitable speed, you need to time your sitting of the CSA for when you have reached the level of 'conscious competence' in GP consulting. 'Conscious competence' means you are performing well, but may need to concentrate in order to do this. For example, as in driving, you may still be needing to *remember* to put the clutch down when you stop the car, but are doing it reliably every time. You may in fact have progressed to unconscious competence in most areas of consulting, the parallel being that it is completely natural to you when to use the clutch and without even thinking. The proviso we would add, of course, is that consulting in general, and specifically in the CSA, is not just about skills but also about knowledge.

The model of development of competence fits more closely to skills than to knowledge, as knowledge is ever changing with new guidelines and medications. Therefore, it is equally as important for you to be assessing your ability in terms of knowledge, constantly updating it and reflecting on whether you are using this knowledge correctly with the patients you see. This will allow you constantly to improve your clinical abilities.

LEARNING POINT 33: Reasons for anticipating difficulty in the CSA

- Self-confidence issues
- Self-reflection
- Timing of exam sitting too early for stage of learning
- Knowledge base
- Clinical and consultation skills
- Health issues

- Life events or work/life balance commitments
- Specific learning difficulties
- Past exam experiences.

Developing effective self-reflection to utilise learning plans

If self-assessment is so unreliable, why do we mention it, especially in the context of trainees having difficulty passing the CSA? Firstly, to lead on to you seeking the honest and constructive assessment from experienced GP trainers or programme directors around you. They will find it much easier to work with you, and to form an effective learning plan for you, if they know your understanding of any issues you may have.

Secondly, most really effective changes in consultation require you to develop insight into what you do that is effective, and what you do that could be improved. In this manner, having agreed areas for development with your experienced educator, you can start by watching videos of your consultations, and spotting those strengths and areas for development. As your self-reflection skills in consulting improve, you should be able to develop this into 'real-time' corrections. For example, during a consultation, you may become able quickly to correct any areas that are not going well in that particular situation. Following on from this, anticipation develops, so that you can avoid encountering such difficulties within the consultation altogether.

What kind of issues may I have if I have not passed the CSA?

This may range from simple to complex, and the solution may vary accordingly. Please, therefore, ask your trainer and programme directors to help confirm whether they agree with your assessment of the likely cause.

Simple causes can include having taken the exam too early in your ST3 year, poor health on the day of the exam or coinciding with some unexpected distraction, for example a sudden life event. If the issue was a one-off, and you can make changes to accommodate the issue, or correct the problem, then progress should be good. We would refer you to the exam preparation chapters earlier in this book. Most importantly, your best practice will be seeing patients, being observed by and observing other experienced GPs in joint surgeries, and also self-reflection on videos of your consultations.

Learning needs

Your reason for not having passed the CSA, the first time, may simply be that there were certain learning needs in terms of knowledge, skills or possibly behaviours (such as negotiation skills, or sharing joint decision making with the patients), which were not quite developed enough on that first occasion. If so, it would be very helpful to go through with your trainer the feedback statements you received with your results, and to refer them to the previous chapter in this book which is a source of helpful pointers as to how you can avoid receiving such feedback statements in the future.

We would like to remind you of the importance of *knowledge* in the CSA exam. It is the experience of many of us as examiners, and also in our roles working with trainees in difficulty, that candidates and trainers usually already recognise the importance of, and work on, developing a good consultation style, but may overlook the level of knowledge needed to pass the CSA. The CSA is designed to test clinical and interpersonal skills. The clinical element has an important influence on the data-gathering domain, and almost complete influence on the clinical management domain. Its influence in data-gathering comes by understanding patterns of symptoms and signs presented, followed by the correct medical understanding of the information elicited, and recommended options for management being offered, individualised to that particular patient in front of you.

Quality of physical examination, when conducted, can also be a common area where marks could be improved. Resources to develop skills in focused, GP-style examination include the link to the section in the national electronic library for health (http://portal.e-lfh.org.uk), or the book '*Pocket Guide to Clinical Examination*', by Epstein et al. (2009). Practise within a 10-minute consultation the types of focused examination which can be conducted in a CSA exam, and this will help you gain those all important marks.

Hence, overall, clinical knowledge and application can give you at least half the marks available in the CSA exam. Examiners on the day, and also the CSA case-writers, all have access to the latest medical guidelines on the condition in question, so committed exploration of the guidance around the range of problems you see in your work as a GP registrar, can prevent very many cases of exam failures, by ensuring you are also well informed.

We hope you would then, together with your trainer, do a CSA PDP (see the Appendix to Chapter 1). One of the important decisions will be how long to wait until the CSA diet you will be sitting. If there is a large improvement needed in scores for you to pass, or a range of feedback areas to tackle, it is helpful to ensure you do not rush into your next attempt, if you have sufficient time left in your training post.

More complex issues

Types of difficulty can include

1 Multiple assessment difficulty (CSA, AKT and WPBA)
2 Specific learning difficulty – for example dyslexia
3 Health difficulty of any type
4 Struggling to prioritise studies due to other commitments
5 Communication or other linguistic difficulties
6 Performance-related difficulties (this can be specific to the CSA, or general performance anxiety).

What types of assessment may I need?

For you to pass the CSA successfully, your needs are most likely to be met if you can openly share your difficulties with your educators. This should not feel like admitting weakness in any way, but should rather feel like a way to access solutions. You should then make contact with the associate director of GP in your region and programme directors to help them input into your new educational plan.

Depending on which of the above difficulties you may have, certain assessments to target help correctly may need to take place. Normally all the types of assessment or help are organised via your patch associate director, or sometimes your programme director.

A *second opinion on your consulting* from one of these senior educators in your patch, seen in combination with the CSA feedback statements you received, would be very important.

If any *specific learning difficulties* are already known, it will help for you to declare them to the RCGP prior to your sitting the exam. The RCGP has a process for considering these to see if any adjustments are needed (such as extra reading time with dyslexia). If it is suspected, but not known, that you may have specific learning difficulty (which can sometimes be more likely in learners struggling with the AKT), an assessment can be arranged via senior educators on your patch.

If you are struggling with *health difficulties*, by discussing these with a senior GP educator, you may need an occupational health assessment. This may result in recommendations, which could help you make the most out of your remaining training. For example, certain adaptations to your working pattern may be suggested if you are exhausted with a medical condition, and hence not able to revise effectively.

Work–life balance issues are likely to be identifiable on open discussion with your trainer, who is probably the educator who knows you best.

If you or your educators feel there may be *communication or linguistic difficulties*, beyond those of GP consultation skills training, it may be helpful to undertake specific linguistic practice in GP consulting. Some regions have access to a language unit, to observe and to help you develop your ability in effective communication with your patients.

The potential for any of us to be misunderstood, or communicate ineffectively, during a GP consultation is enormous. This was recently brought home in a patient letter, where the patient understood fully the words used, even repeating them in the letter, but had completely misunderstood the intention of those words. If, having been a GP for more than 20 years, knowing the patient, and not being under the stress of an exam, one of us can find ourselves in this position; there is certainly a risk of this for any candidate in the exam.

Any techniques which can help us identify where our phrasing could be ambiguous, with suggestions for improvement, must surely be welcome. In addition, one of the intentions of writing this book is to ensure that all candidates can have insight into help and support which would put them in the best possible position for passing the exam.

Performance anxiety, if impacting on your performance, may need assessment by a psychologist, who would also recommend treatments and strategies. Different areas of the country have different providers for this. For example, in London Mednet and also the practitioner health programme are available, which can assess and provide treatment. Wherever you reside, your associate director of GP will be able to signpost you, or refer you to appropriate resources after assessing your situation.

What types of help and solutions are available for me?

Treatments or *strategies* for those difficulties mentioned above are likely to follow on from assessment. This would be in addition to you making use of the suggestions for all candidates in the earlier chapters.

Multiple assessment failures (AKT/CSA/WPBA) would need a detailed educational plan in conjunction with your associate director in GP following the assessments detailed earlier. This would include plans regarding timescale, and any extension to GP training that is felt to be needed if you have reached the end of ST3. The more complex the issues, the more likely it is that reducing your working percentage to less than full time will be advantageous educationally. This will give you a longer time before you have to re-sit the exams and also allow more time every week for you to read, reflect and practise your consulting with peers.

If a *specific learning difficulty* of any type is diagnosed, the specialist educational unit making this diagnosis will be able to assist with strategies to prevent this affecting your learning during training and your performance during the exam.

If you have *health difficulties*, specific occupational health advice for you, as well as ensuring that you are seeking medical help, will be very important. Again, in some cases, you may feel, with your associate director, that reducing your percentage to less than full-time training may assist you educationally, or accessing additional medical help may resolve the effect of your condition on exam performance.

Work–life balance issues may find solutions within your wider network of family and friends. Letting them know that you are struggling, and that you really need any practical help with your home commitments until you have passed the CSA may help. You may find, if home is very hectic, that identifying suitable times and places to study or practise will be important. Some geographical areas also have 'mentoring' available for learners which can help equip you with the tools to manage your complex and conflicting demands in a way that helps your exam chances.

Consultation skills: Joint surgeries with experienced educators and also observing experienced educators consulting are extremely helpful. Please see if you can build this into your educational half-days. Videoing and assessing the recordings yourself (using the feedback statements and information on the RCGP website as to what the examiners are looking for) will be helpful. Please also see the previous chapter on how not to get the feedback statements. Practising with other learners is also very useful, *but beware of always practising with others who did not pass the CSA first time, as you may reinforce each other's behaviours which were noted on the first sitting.*

Regarding *performance-related difficulties*, for mild anxiety, a range of strategies can help, including those mentioned in the first chapter on 'maximizing performance'. However, if you feel, following assessment, that performance anxiety is sufficient to affect your success in the CSA, we would encourage you to access cognitive behavioural therapy. For many registrars, this has paid dividends.

LEARNING POINT 34: Strategies for Improvement

- Strategies from experienced educators into your educational plan
- Develop effective self-reflection

- Specialised help for learning or health issues
- Consultation skills and linguistic resources
- Psychological resources.

Conclusion

Most importantly, try not to feel alone if you have not passed the CSA first time. Please try to access all the support you can get from educators, peers, friends and family. By doing this, you can walk into the exam next time more confidently, having made maximum use of all these strategies and your support networks.

References

Electronic library for health – http://portal.e-lfh.org.uk, register or log in. Choose launch health management system, then e GP 00 introductory guides, then 00_04 Guide to physical examination.

Epstein, O., et al. (2009) "Pocket Guide to Clinical Examination" Published by Mosby, London, 4th edition, updated May 2009, ISBN: 13: 9781563756115, http://www.amazon.co.uk/Pocket-Guide-Clinical-Examination-Mosby/dp/0723434654#reader_0723434654.

Chapter 8 **Learning points**

The following is a collation of the essential learning points from the earlier chapters.

LEARNING POINT 1: 'My CSA PDP' – resources for improvement

- RCGP e-modules EKU (Essential Knowledge Updates) are compiled by representatives of the examiners' panel.
- 'Innovait' – covers every section of the Curriculum on a 3 yearly cycle (ST1-3).
- Summaries of GP guidelines such as 'e-guidelines' which also produce a book with a compilation of current guidance in handy flow charts and tables.
- GP free magazines which include CPD or review articles, for example 'Prescriber' magazine.
- 'PUNs and DENs' after each surgery, with a quick reference to the current guidelines after seeing patients.

LEARNING POINT 2: Examiners' feedback statements – areas commonly highlighted by examiners as needing improvement

- Consultation structure/time management.
- Management plans in keeping with current best practice.
- Identifying the patient's agenda, health beliefs and preferences.
- Use of verbal and non-verbal cues. Active listening.
- Sharing the management plan, clarifying the roles of doctor and patient (RCGP, 2014; Trafford, 2010).

The CSA Exam: Maximizing your Success, First Edition. Rachel Roberts.

Companion Website: www.wiley.com\go\Roberts\CSAExam

LEARNING POINT 3: Tips for effective consulting style in the CSA

- Become interested and curious.
- Create rapport.
- Ask questions.
- *Listen* and check your understanding of what the patient describes.
- Pay particular attention to the patient's non-verbal communication.

LEARNING POINT 4: Performance management tips

- Replace unhelpful, negative thinking with positive thoughts.
- Replace your concerns about your perceived weaknesses with tools to overcome them.
- Act calmly.
- Be aware of your own body language and non-verbal cues.
- When the buzzer ends the consultation in the CSA, clear your head for the next case.

LEARNING POINT 5: Verbalise your thoughts

Examiners can't read your mind! It is essential throughout the exam that you verbalise your thought process for the examiner to hear and mark.

LEARNING POINT 6: Active listening [1]

As well as just listening, *your* body language, eye contact and demeanour are all essential in making the patient want to talk and open up to you.

LEARNING POINT 7: Active listening [2]

Remember that the role-player has been primed to 'cue' you, so listen to what you are being told and watch for non-verbal cues. For the first minute or so of the consultation try to say as little as possible yourself, just using positive body language and open questions or phrases to encourage the 'patient' to open up to you.

LEARNING POINT 8: Active listening [3]
'Tell me more' may simply lead to the 'patient' replying 'What do you want to know?' So try to make the question more specific – for example 'Tell me when they (headaches) start'.

LEARNING POINT 9: Active listening [4]
Listen and reflect explicitly – 'You said earlier … '; 'Did I hear you say … '

LEARNING POINT 10: Hidden agendas
If there *is* a hidden agenda, the clues for you will usually be in the body language, lack of eye contact, slow or distracted speech.

LEARNING POINT 11: Why candidates may fail on interpersonal skills
A candidate who fails on interpersonal skills

- Does not use positive body language and eye contact to encourage the patient to talk
- Does not listen and then respond to what the patient is saying
- Does not respond to cues – verbal or non-verbal – given by the patient
- Shows a lack of genuine interest by talking over or lecturing the patient
- Is not genuinely empathetic towards the patient
- Does not interact with the patient as in a proper conversation
- Does not involve the patient in the diagnosis or clinical management
- Ticks the boxes of his/her own agenda, asking questions by rote, no matter what the patient is saying
- Uses Social, Psycho-social, Ideas, Concerns and Expectations (SPICE) questions insensitively and inappropriately
- Does not get to the point, or fails to comprehend the patient's agenda
- Does not understand the impact of the problem on the patient's life, family, work and so on.
- Offers leaflets, not explanations (examiners cannot mark leaflets!)

LEARNING POINT 12: Structure your consultation

You need to have a clear structure in mind for your consultation, and to remember to include the 'patient' by sharing ideas, options and decisions throughout.

LEARNING POINT 13: Physical Examination 1

If it is appropriate to examine on a day-to-day basis in your surgery, then it is appropriate to do so in the CSA – and to do it properly because your technique will be assessed!

LEARNING POINT 14: Physical examination 2

Think about the scenarios entailing actual physical examination – joints, for example – which are likely to occur in the CSA, and watch videos of good practice for such examinations.

LEARNING POINT 15: Timing the consultation

Don't spend too much time on the data-gathering to the detriment of management! Many candidates fail because of an inadequate or inappropriate management plan.

LEARNING POINT 16: Gender balance

Half of each day's CSA cases will be male, the other half female. How much exposure do you get in your day-to-day surgery dealing with both genders? Male trainees, for example, often don't see the gynaecology or contraception cases.

LEARNING POINT 17: The 'angry patient' 1

One of the cases you encounter in the CSA may involve an 'angry patient'. The crucial thing to remember here is that you have never met the person before, so they can never actually be angry at you – but at some incident. Apologising *for the situation the person finds themselves in* as early as possible in the consultation (without making judgements or taking sides) will diffuse much of the anger.

LEARNING POINT 18: The 'angry patient' 2

Remember to keep calm, not to mirror the angry person's speech patterns, tone of voice or body language. Such cases are always difficult, but remind yourself that everyone doing the exam on that day will also have to deal with it and will find it equally hard.

LEARNING POINT 19: Be yourself!

In the CSA you should be your normal, doctoring self. The CSA is simply examining good general practice, so don't try to act any differently from the way you are on a day-to-day basis, or – put another way – act the way you do in the CSA in your normal life as a GP, and you won't go wrong.

LEARNING POINT 20: Read the patient records

It is good practice to spend 2 minutes looking at the summary patient records – medications and last consultation, relevant recent results, correspondence (the kind of information generally gleaned from good housekeeping). In this sense, you are already gathering data and increasing your likelihood of having an efficient and effective consultation and setting the tone of your greeting – a great habit to get into not just for the CSA but also for your life as a GP.

LEARNING POINT 21: A CSA-style appointments schedule template

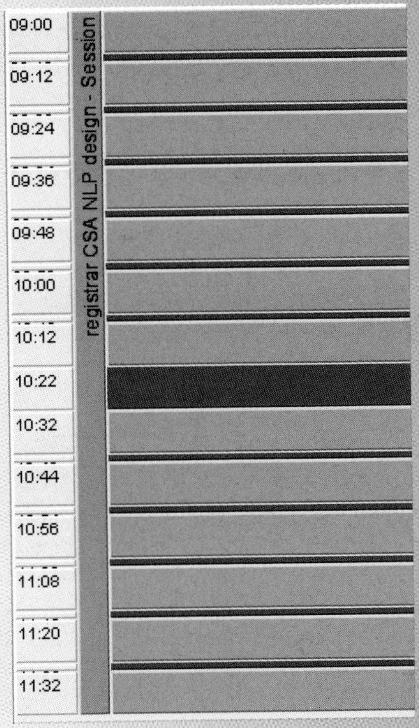

LEARNING POINT 22: Observers

Don't be alarmed if, during your CSA exam, more than one apparent 'assessor' enters the room. There are often 'occasional others'. These may include Quality Assurance personnel who are monitoring the role-players, or visiting dignitaries, lay observers, observers from other colleges, or interested bodies such as the CQC and GP schools representatives.

LEARNING POINT 23: Time-keeping

It is worth recreating the time-up clock in your own consulting room to give yourself a feel for exam conditions, and it will help you manage consultation time more effectively. By getting a 'feel' for what a 5-minute span is like, you will know when to start to move into the clinical management stage of a 10-minute consultation.

LEARNING POINT 24: Data-gathering

The first 'cue' you get about each patient in the CSA is the information written in the patient records. So start your data-gathering for each case as soon as possible.

LEARNING POINT 25: The pivot point

In terms of exam technique, utilising the examination phase of a case as a *pivot point* to move on from the Data-Gathering phase into the Clinical Management phase may be helpful. While the patient is getting themselves back together is a good time for you to confidently open up a discussion about diagnosis and management – for example

'Did you have any thoughts about what is going on here and what we might do about it?' ('not really, doctor') … 'having listened to what you have said, and examined you carefully, what I think is … what do you think?'

LEARNING POINT 26: Clinical management

The Clinical Management domain is where most marks are lost – often because of time lost in the Data-Gathering phase. Most candidates do the history-taking really well and do it confidently. But the danger is that it becomes a comfort zone they don't want to leave! *Generally speaking* you should be getting into the Clinical Management zone by 6 minutes, and you need to have the competence and confidence to be moving the consultation on without appearing to rush by that time.

LEARNING POINT 27: Re-calling the patient

If a consultation ends before the 10 minutes are up the patient may leave. If, however, you then suddenly realise you want to cover something else or to correct an aspect of your management, it is absolutely fine within the 10 minutes allowed for the case, to retrieve your patient from the 'waiting room'. Role-players and examiners are under strict instruction to wait outside your door and your marks will not be given until the 10-minute buzzer sounds. This might make a difference to your marks if, for example, you show that you recognise you have recommended an inappropriate drug (allergy?/interaction?).

LEARNING POINT 28: The 2 minutes between cases

Ctrl + Alt + Delete

Take a deep breath and use the 2-minute break for 'housekeeping'. Clear your mind of the previous case – even if you think you have messed it up, don't waste time agonising about what you should or shouldn't have done! The chances are you did better than you think anyway!
So, 'Control/Alt/Delete'! Regain your composure and move on to look at the records of the next case. Start data-gathering again.

LEARNING POINT 29: Upon what values do we base our decisions?

This is not an exhaustive list of underlying VALUES. However, it may help dissect and direct the solving of dilemmas:

- Professional values, for example GMC guidelines/Good medical practice
- Evidence-based medicine, for example NICE and other guidelines
- Legal values – the laws of the country
- Cultural and religious values
- International law
- Moral convictions

LEARNING POINT 30: Go back to your e-portfolio

Look at compliments/SEAs/complaints.

Reflect on them and ask what can be learnt from them ... and how that learning might be tested in a CSA case?

LEARNING POINT 31: So, what sort of questions should you be asking yourself?

Every consultation has implicit ethical issues, but you must be aware of, and be prepared to discuss, the explicit issues.

- Is your appointment system too easy or too difficult to access?
- Is your hospital over- or under-treating?
- What is the balance in the decision making in your CCG – patient care versus balancing budget ... what are your attitudes, those of colleagues, those of your trainer, partners, salaried, examiners, ... how and what might make these change over time ... and with reducing resources?

LEARNING POINT 32: First steps in addressing candidate concerns

- Identify potential barriers to success
- Develop self awareness
- Enlist appropriate help
- Develop appropriate strategies
- Be aware of available resources

LEARNING POINT 33: Reasons for anticipating difficulty in the CSA

- Self -confidence issues
- Self-reflection
- Timing of exam sitting – too early for stage of learning
- Knowledge base
- Clinical and consultation skills
- Health issues
- Life events or work/life balance commitments
- Specific learning difficulties
- Past exam experiences

LEARNING POINT 34: Strategies for improvement for the CSA

- Strategies from experienced educators into your educational plan
- Develop effective self-reflection
- Specialised help for learning or health issues
- Consultation skills and linguistic resources
- Psychological resources

Part Two

A 'palette' of 16 CSA-type cases and 6 ethical cases

'The first 12 cases, marked with a "V", are available as video clips on the website which accompanies the book'.

Clips of cases two, nine and twelve show examples of the full 10 minute CSA consultation.

Please note that clips of the other nine cases have been filmed as an introduction to the case and for you to question what you might do next in this consultation. They are NOT intended as examples of a full CSA consultation.

Taking the opportunity to take over the role-play in pairs or in groups, from that point on is ideal, then using the questions and marking schedules to critically assess your consultation.

The final four cases on the list marked [P] are examples of the types of the recently introduced paediatric cases involving child actors which you may encounter in the CSA.

The remaining 6 video clips are of ethical dilemmas for you in pairs or groups to practise taking up the role play from where the clip ends. Hence you will practise managing difficult ethical dilemmas in preparation for the CSA. Supporting material for those cases is found in chapter 4, dealing with challenging situations.

7	Jenny Stanley	[V]
8	Harry Evans	[V]
9	Shona Baker	[V]
10	Amelia Kowalski	[V]
11	Thomas Smith	[V]
12	Debbie Wells	[V]
13	Ashia Pollock	[P]
14	Olu Wa-Simba	[P]
15	Nilesh Patel	[P]
16	Stephanie Caldwell	[P]

Introduction to the sample cases

The following pages contain 16 sample CSA cases for you to practise in pairs or in small groups. For each scenario, you will need to decide who is to be the 'Candidate/Doctor' and who is to role-play the 'Simulated Patient'. If there are more than two of you participating, any others should act as 'Assessors/Examiners'.

The layout of each case is similar, with separate sections for the different participants.

Thus, the first couple of pages outline what the '*Patient*' needs to know, that is,

- Name, age and background
- An opening statement
- Information to give
- Information to give if asked specifically by the doctor
- Questions to ask the doctor if appropriate
- Behaviour/demeanour/body language

There will also be some Notes for preparing to role-play the case, which may include instructions for an '*Examiner*'.

A couple of points:

1 The person who is to be the doctor in the consultation should not read these pages beforehand.
2 The 'Patient' must remember that they are the 'uninformed patient' and should question jargon or medical terminology which a lay person would not understand.
3 Don't give all the information away at once. Expect the 'Doctor' to tease it out of you.

The CSA Exam: Maximizing your Success, First Edition. Rachel Roberts.

Companion Website: www.wiley.com\go\Roberts\CSAExam

4 Role-playing is different from acting. It is important to play the 'Patient' as naturally and realistically as possible. Try to get inside the head of this 'patient' and understand their SPICE (*S*ocial and *P*sycho-social background, *I*deas, *C*oncerns and *E*xpectations).

The '*Candidate/Doctor*' should be allowed up to 2 minutes to read the case notes for the 'Patient'. The materials for the doctor which, in the CSA, will be displayed on the iPad usually consist of the following:

- Patient's Name, Age and Address
- Social and Family History
- Past Medical History
- Current Medication
- Other Clinical Details

If there are other members of the study group observing, they should act as 'Examiners'.

If the case being practised entails *actual physical examination*

- Are the people practising the case comfortable with being examined?

If so, this allows correct practice of the case, including feedback on examination choices and technique. These are areas where candidates can lose marks, so it is well worth practising.

- If those practising are not comfortable with being examined, please decide before role-playing the case how you will deal with this.

If physical examination is undertaken, assuming it is done properly and in a manner which would elicit findings, then the results of the examination should be given by an 'Examiner' – either by producing the 'Examination Card' included in the case paperwork or by giving the findings verbally.

If there is no 'Examiner', then the 'Patient' should give the card or the verbal findings.

Please note, however, that the findings given must also be appropriate to the physical examination offered by the 'Candidate'; that is, if the doctor does not ask to take the 'patient's' blood pressure, and that is on the 'Examination Card', then that finding should NOT be given.

'*Examiners*' should also read the 'Case Marking Sheet', which outlines what the case-writer expects as positive (or possibly negative) behaviours in the three domains of

- Data-Gathering
- Clinical Management
- Interpersonal Skills

The 'Examiners' should watch the role-played consultation closely and make notes of what they hear and observe, so that they can give feedback afterwards with *specific examples* of good behaviour – or what might be improved – referring to the descriptors in the marking sheet.

When giving feedback, remember Pendleton rules! Discuss what went well, before launching into what might be improved upon or done differently!

- Ask the 'Candidate' what went well
- Ask the observers what went well
- Ask the 'Patient' how it felt for him/her
- Only now, start to discuss what might be done differently.

If one of the observers suggests a different approach, then role-play that immediately with the 'Patient' and see if it alters the outcome.

The final page of each case scenario contains explanations from the case-writer as to what the case is intended to test, and some suggestions for learning resources to use as follow-up.

We hope you find the following cases useful as practice for the CSA.

Case 1

Name of 'Patient': **Alan Arterton**
Gender: Male
Age: 35

Background

- You work as a land surveyor
- You are happily married
- You have two children, aged 8 and 9 – all well

Opening statement

'Doc, I am having to go to the toilet a lot'

(slightly embarrassed)

Information to give if specifically asked

- You have to open your bowels more frequently over the last few months (if asked – 6 months).
- Your normal bowel habit was once a day – now it's two or three times a day.
- It is not loose nor diarrhoea, and there is no blood or mucous.
- You have no abdominal pain, no vomiting or bloating.
- You have lost about half a stone in weight over 6 months, but you put this down to slightly healthier eating and perhaps a little more walking in the job.
- Your healthy eating is because you're 35, and it won't be long before your 40th birthday, hence you want to stay healthy.
- If asked whether you have any other symptoms, you have noticed a tremor in your hands in the last few months.

The CSA Exam: Maximizing your Success, First Edition. Rachel Roberts.

Companion Website: www.wiley.com\go\Roberts\CSAExam

If asked about other symptoms, ask the doctor what sort of symptoms?

- You have noticed you get sweaty much easier than before 6 months ago.
- You have not noticed any palpitations (fast heartbeat).
- No change in urine habit.
- No change in skin.

If asked how this is impacting on work and home life?

- It is sometimes embarrassing when you are surveying on different building sites, you have to use the builders' portaloos and you now know where the public toilets are on various train stations.

IDEA – your bowel habit changes are related to diet.
CONCERN – you have a minor doubt in your mind because some of your relatives in Ireland have got coeliac disease, but not the immediate family, and you thought you might have this.
EXPECTATION – you are hoping to have tests to find the cause and possibly exclude coeliac disease.

Past medical history

- Age 17 – appendectomy
- No change at work – no stress been used to job with the same firm since University
- Smoker – 10 a day since aged 16
- Alcohol social – (if pushed, no more than 1 glass of wine, 2 or 3 days a week)
- Family history – nil all well mainly in Ireland – HOWEVER only if asked.

Expect the candidate to ask to examine you

You will be expected to let the doctor take your pulse.
They may ask you to hold your arms outstretched. If so, please create a slight tremor the fingers.
They may want to gently palpate the thyroid gland that is located in the front of your neck.
They may want to examine your eyes – and in this case please follow their instructions.
If they ask to examine your tummy or your blood pressure or your weight, the examiner will intervene and give them the information card.

Questions for the role-player to ask the doctor, if appropriate

'Is this dangerous doctor?'

If the doctor decides you may have something seriously wrong with your bowels and you need to be referred urgently, you will look worried and half-heartedly try to reassure the doctor and yourself perhaps this is not serious because it has been going on for 6 months.

If the doctor suggests this is related to diet or irritable bowel syndrome, you will accept their diagnosis and ask how to manage it?

If the doctor suggests this is a thyroid problem, you will look surprised as you thought thyroid problems only occurred in older people?

If the doctor says you need any blood tests – you will ask what blood test the doctor is going to order and why?

'How will this be treated?'

We would expect the doctor to explain all your symptoms being related to the thyroid and explain this can be easily treated with a drug called carbimazole, if blood test confirms thyrotoxicosis. You should ask how long you will need this drug.

'What are the side effects of this drug?'

The doctor may explain you will need regular blood tests with this medication and you will accept this without any concern. The doctor may also explain that, while on these tablets, if you have a sore throat, rash fever or malaise, you should contact the doctors immediately for a blood test.

You will also ask 'Will I need this medication all my life and is there any other treatment?'

You may need this treatment long term, however. The doctor may discuss the possibility of an ultrasound scan as an investigation. This may show a hot nodule in the thyroid and this may need an operation, in this case you will not look worried but pleased that it can be easily sorted rather than taking tablets for a long period.

You may need referral to a specialist called an Endocrinologist and you are happy to accept this.

Behaviour/demeanour/body language

Calm, co-operative and accepts doctor's recommendations.

If a 2-week-wait referral to the bowel specialist is suggested, then you become anxious. You then try to question the doctor as to whether a serious condition would have persisted for 6 months.

Issues for preparation of the case

- Instructions to the person playing the 'Examiner':

If the candidate suggests they want to examine the pulse, eyes and thyroid, they should be told to do so. After the examination has been completed in a proper manner, please offer the card or give the findings verbally appropriate to the examination undertaken.

If only two people are doing the role-play, the 'Patient' will give the card, or give the findings verbally appropriate to the examination undertaken

If the candidate suggests examining anything else, state that those findings are 'normal'.

Examination Card

Candidate expected to examine – thyroid, eyes, outstretched hands

- Pulse 94 SR
- Apyrexial
- BP 134/80
- Weight 65 kg
- Thyroid exam normal
- Eye exam normal

Materials for the doctor [displayed on the iPad in the CSA]

Case notes for the patient

Name:	Alan Arterton
Age:	35
Address:	4 Calder Drive

Social and family history

- Land surveyor

Past medical history

- Age 17 – appendectomy

Current medication

Nil

CSA Case Marking Sheet: Case name: Alan Arterton [Case 1]	
Focus for the case: Testing the candidate's ability to manage a young man with increased bowel frequency and weight loss. Arranging suitable treatment and management	
Data-gathering, technical and assessment skills	• Take a systematic history to exclude other bowel pathology • Do a targeted examination and investigation. Avoid overinvestigation
Positive descriptors: • History elucidates 6-month history and weight loss • Focused history to exclude other causes and red flag symptoms • Explores family history • Examination is focused to include thyroid, eyes, pulse, and weight • Good candidate picks up family history and impact on work	**Negative descriptors:** • Disorganised gathering of data which does not appear guided by probabilities of disease • Focuses narrowly on the problem, for example only concentrating on diarrhoea and weight loss with no exploration of any other potential symptoms or causes • Examination does not include the relevant focused elements or is conducted with poor technique
Clinical Management skills	Manage symptoms, possible medication after tests and refer appropriately
Positive descriptors: • Recognises the significance of the symptoms and explains thyrotoxicosis • Safe discussion of carbimazole prescription • Explains endocrine referral and long-term management of thyrotoxicosis and possible hospital interventions • Manages some health promotion to quit smoking • Follow-up by GP explained	**Negative descriptors:** • Candidate does not appear to reach appropriate differential diagnoses • Management is not conducted with appropriate referral • Follow-up arrangements either at hospital or GP not mentioned • Candidate does not mention safe prescribing of carbimazole

Interpersonal skills	Explain the diagnosis and explore concerns
Positive descriptors: • Active listening and appropriately responds to problem without alarming the patient • Provides relevant explanation of possible link of change in bowel habit and weight loss with thyrotoxicosis • Explains coeliac's disease and the test to exclude this diagnosis • Maintains warmth and understanding while exploring the symptoms and possible causes	**Negative descriptors:** • Poor active listening skills • Causes unnecessary anxiety in the patient • Explanations of potential causes are not relevant or appropriate to the patient • Manner lacks warmth and understanding

Name of the 'Patient':	**Alan Arterton** [Case 1]
Curriculum Clinical Statement:	3.17 Care of People with Metabolic Problems

This case is testing the candidate's ability to

- Take a systematic history to exclude other bowel pathology.
- Do a targeted examination and investigation. Avoid overinvestigation.
- Explain the diagnosis and explore concerns.
- Manage symptoms, possible medication after tests and refer appropriately.

Learning resources

http://www.patient.co.uk/doctor/hyperthyroidism.

http://learning.bmj.com/learning/module-intro/hyperthyroidism--diagnosis-and-treatment.html?moduleId=5003139.

http://bestpractice.bmj.com/best-practice/evidence/background/0611.html.

Case 2

Name of 'Patient': **Jane Smith re Isabel Chalk**
Gender: Female
Age: 72 (phoning about your friend, Isabel, also aged 72)

Background

- You are phoning the doctor today as you are very worried about your friend, Isabel Chalk, who is aged 72.
- You have known Isabel since you both went to art college together 50 or more years ago.
- You now live in the Isle of Wight and visit Isabel around once a month.
- Isabel lives alone and was widowed 2 years ago.
- She lives in an affluent suburban area in a detached house.
- She has a lifelong interest in art and has written several books on the subject.
- She has no children.
- Her husband was a solicitor who had retired before dying of lung cancer 2 years ago.

Opening statement

'I hope you can help doctor. I'm phoning you about my friend Isabel. I'm really worried about her'

(delivered in a concerned tone of voice, but friendly and open)

The CSA Exam: Maximizing your Success, First Edition. Rachel Roberts.

Companion Website: www.wiley.com\go\Roberts\CSAExam

Information to give

Secondary statement – *'I was visiting her last week and every time I visit, she seems to be neglecting herself more and more'.*

- You are worried by a number of areas of your friend's behaviour recently and believe alcohol to be the cause.
- Isabel often seems to be unable to answer the phone or come to the door to let you in, having forgotten that you're due to see her.
- When you are together, you notice that she drinks alcohol or has already been drinking when you arrive and she looks unwell.
- There often does not seem to be enough food in the house and her clothes appear dirty, which is completely out of character for her.
- In the last year and a half she's had a few accidents within the house: on one occasion breaking her wrist and on the second occasion dislocating her shoulder
- You are suspicious that alcohol played a part in both of these incidents. The hospital did not seem to pick up on this, and she was sent straight home after treating the injury.
- If asked to arrange an appointment for her to come and see the doctor, or for the doctor to visit, then explain that Isabel gets very angry and upset when asked to see the doctor and denies any health problems or excessive alcohol drinking
- You have tried very hard to persuade her already over several months to see the doctor but have failed so far.
- You do know, however, that she's got on well with the doctors from this practice and are hopeful that, if you meet face-to-face, she would accept help.
- She has no remaining family but you are one of two friends (Susan is the other) who live far away and visit every 3–4 weeks separately.
- She does have supportive neighbours and you're aware that her neighbour has a key to her house and you're hoping that the doctor will agree to visit Isabel, asking the neighbour to let you in if she doesn't answer the door.
- If the candidate asks questions to try and ascertain the seriousness of her health problems, please give the following information:
  Isabel seems to be getting much worse and, this time when you visited her, her eyes looked very yellow. Her face appears puffy, and there were signs that she had been incontinent of urine on some of the furniture and in the bedroom.
- She does seem to understand and be able to make decisions when you ask her what she would like to do, but does not seem interested in helping herself and appears to have given up.

- If the doctor says they cannot discuss her with you and, therefore, does not try to ask you for any information, you can become rather distressed. If this occurs, please ask the doctor what they are going to do to help your friend.
- If they say they cannot discuss her further with you but will arrange to visit, please ask that they contact you to let you know what's happening as you're so worried.
- Explain that one of the salaried doctors did visit 2 months ago but that she refused all treatments and you are no further forward. This was following a previous phone call you made to the practice to express your worries.
- You are not able to return for another month due to family commitments (your husband is not at all well with Parkinson's disease), and neither is your friend Susan.

Questions to ask the doctor, if appropriate

Whether the doctor has a detailed discussion with you, or whether they decline to speak to you at all about her, please ask

- 'What will you do if you see Isabel and she refuses any treatment?'
- 'What will you do if you visit and she doesn't open the door – I really feel she is very unwell'
- 'GP visited her 2 months ago and said she had an alcohol problem giving her lots of vitamins and a number for her to ring to see someone but she just didn't go – what can you do now?'

Behaviour/demeanour/body language

Your tone is concerned and co-operative but, if you feel nothing is going to be done, you will be persistent. You are concerned enough to feel your friend may even die if no help is provided and, therefore, are prepared to insist on some action being taken.

Issues for Preparation of the Case

Telephone triage consultations are best practised with the 'Patient' and doctor sitting back-to-back so that non-verbal cues are not apparent.

Materials for the doctor [displayed on the iPad in the CSA]

Case notes for the patient

Name:	**Isabel Chalk** (her friend, Jane Smith, is phoning you)
Age:	72
Address:	10 Tavistock Close

Social and family history

- Retired author on art
- Widowed

Past medical history

- 18 months ago – colles fracture left wrist after a fall in the house
- 2 months ago – dislocation of the right shoulder after a fall.

Current medication

- 2 months ago
- Thiamine 100 mg twice daily ×56
- Vitamin B complex strong twice daily ×56
- Omeprazole 20 mg ×28
- None collected since

Other clinical details

- Visit 2 months ago by Dr Smith after call from a concerned friend.
- Signs of chronic alcoholism, number for alcohol team given, referral for mental health assessment, commenced thiamine, vitamin B complex strong and omeprazole.
- 6 weeks ago, letter back from mental health team, 'Mrs Chalk declined our offer of an assessment, so we have closed her case.'

CSA Case Marking Sheet: Case name: Isabel Chalk [Case 2]	
Focus for case: Deal with a complex ethical dilemma when significant medical problems may be present. Sensitive management in relation to a patient with significant alcohol problems.	
Data-gathering, technical and assessment skills	Gathers data regarding problem drinking and the reported state of health in a hard-to-reach patient
Positive descriptors: • Takes a detailed history from the friend regarding the background • History ascertains the seriousness of the physical signs of the effects of alcohol • History ascertains concerns about depression and precipitant of being widowed • Candidate appreciates the lack of progress after attempt at interventions 2 months ago	**Negative descriptors:** • Candidate declines to take information from the friend regarding Isabel • Does not ascertain the seriousness of the physical health problem • Does not enquire regarding mood effect of widowhood or social support
Clinical Management skills	Works within ethical boundaries to find a way forward to assess the patient effectively

Positive descriptors: • Finds a workable solution to allow the patient to be assessed • Addresses friend's concerns, while working within ethical boundaries of patient • Shows an understanding of the need to balance respect for patient autonomy, with the risk to life, and need to assess her capacity • Considers the possibility that mental state and capacity need formal assessment • Understands the teams available to support patients with alcohol, mental health and also physical issues • Understands that there may be a need for social services input	**Negative descriptors:** • Makes immediate assumptions that cannot assess information or seriousness of the problem by receiving information from the friend • Candidate does not show flexibility in problem solving • Candidate struggles to manage the ethical aspects of this case • Breaks patient confidentiality by revealing any patient information not volunteered by the friend • Fails to understand the vulnerability of the patient and the possible need for social services involvement • Fails to understand the need to assess the patient's mental state
Interpersonal skills	Shows respect for the friend, and concern for the patient, while working within ethical boundaries
Positive descriptors: • Active listening to understand the extent of the problem • Sympathetic to the concerns of the friend • Persistent in trying to find a workable solution • Communication shows a respect for the patient herself	**Negative descriptors:** • Poor listening to friend's concerns • Candidate seems uncomfortable, affecting empathy or shared management • Candidate appears judgemental • Candidate is not able to show shared negotiation in the telephone consultation

Name of the patient: **Isabel Chalk** [Case 2]
Curriculum Clinical Statement: 3.14 – Care of people who misuse drugs and alcohol

This case is testing the candidate's ability to

- Deal with a complex ethical dilemma when significant medical problems may be present
- Get a detailed history regarding the extent of the friend's clinical concern
- Try to find a workable solution whereby the patient could access medical help and an assessment
- Show ability to use ethical frameworks practically, while addressing this complex problem.

Learning resources

National Institute for Health and Clinical Excellence (NICE). Alcohol-use disorders: diagnosis, assessment and management of harmful drinking and alcohol dependence, National Institute for Health and Clinical Excellence (NICE) Clinical Guideline CG 115 February 2011.

Also NICE guidelines learning resource. http://www.alcohollearningcentre.org.uk/Topics/Browse/Commissioning/PbR/NICEGuidelines/.

RCGP e-courses. RCGP Management of Alcohol Problems in Primary Care. www.alcoholics-anonymous.org.uk. Resources for patients and doctors.

Case 3

Name of 'Patient': **Jason Brown**
Gender: Male
Age: 52

Background

- Works as a telephone operator in a call centre
- Divorced 5 years ago, with two grown-up children from that marriage
- Lives with his partner Jane the last 3 years.

Opening statement

'Have you got the results of my X-ray please, doctor?'

Information to give

- You started to cough around 7 or 8 weeks ago. When you walk fast or try to walk up a hill you become breathless.
- You have had two courses of antibiotics from the doctor during this time and do not feel any better.
- You smoked 20 cigarettes a day but gave up around 20 years ago.
- You drink around 4 pints of beer a week, to socialise with friends in the pub.
- You have had some clear to white phlegm persistently for the 7 or 8 weeks. It can seem a little runny in consistency at times.
- You have not noticed any blood when you cough.
- You've had no temperatures.

The CSA Exam: Maximizing your Success, First Edition. Rachel Roberts.

Companion Website: www.wiley.com\go\Roberts\CSAExam

- You have no pain when you try and exert yourself, although you are breathless.
- You have no palpitations, and no other symptoms.

Information to give, if asked specifically by the doctor

- You are breathless at night recently and have had to use three pillows in bed, as it is worse if you're lying flat.
- Your father had a heart attack at the age of 54, but then lived on until 70, when he died of another heart attack.
- You have been seeing a nurse regularly for weight management and orlistat from 18 months ago until 3 months ago.
- The weight tablets you were having worked at first, but when you had had no improvement in the last 6 months they had been stopped. Since then your weight has rocketed, and you have lost all motivation.
- *Your weight is currently 26 stone 2 lb.*
- Your diet does include some fried food, and you tend to miss breakfast, and then start snacking on biscuits at work. You do try hard, but dislike fruit and vegetables. You like sausages and pies.
- Your job is sedentary; you have tried to add walking regularly when on orlistat, but have now lost all motivation since stopping this tablet.

Questions to ask the doctor, if appropriate

- 'Is it the chest infection I've had which has caused this fluid on the lung/heart failure?' (depending which term the doctor uses)
- If offered tablets – 'So how long is this course of tablets, doctor?'
- 'So can't you cure this problem at all?'
- 'Why has this happened to me?'
- 'Could my heart stop doctor?'

Behaviour/demeanour/body language

Initial opening statement fairly relaxed, but becoming concerned as the news is broken.

You are willing to accept any tests or treatment offered by the doctor, but you do not really grasp at first that this is a long-term problem.

Physical examination

Expect the doctor to ask to examine you. If this happens, ask what they would like to examine. Expect to have your arm free to be checked for pulse and blood pressure, to have your chest checked with a stethoscope and your ankles to be checked. They may also look at your neck for jugulovenous pressure.

Issues for preparation of the case

- Instructions to the person playing the 'Examiner':

  After examination has been completed, please offer the card or give the findings verbally appropriate to the examination undertaken.

  If only two people are doing the role-play, the 'Patient' will give the card, or give the findings verbally appropriate to the examination undertaken.

Examination Card

- Pulse 84 and regular
- BP 180/90
- Jugulovenous pressure raised 2 cm
- Normal heart sounds
- Lung fields, very few fine inspiratory crepitations at the bases
- Mild-to-moderate ankle swelling symmetrically

Materials for the doctor [displayed on the iPad in the CSA]

Case notes for the patient

Name:	Jason Brown
Age:	52
Address:	25 Stoneleigh Road

Social and family history

- Works in a call centre full time
- Divorced 5 years ago; has two adult children
- Last 3 years lives with his partner Jane.

Past medical history

- Nurse appointments starting 18 months ago and lasting till 3 months ago for orlistat.
  Body mass index over 50.
- Orlistat was initially effective, but no weight loss in the last 6 months; hence, medication was discontinued 3 months ago.
- Ex-smoker, stopped 20 years ago.
- 5 weeks ago seen with cough, felt to be chest infection, prescribed amoxicillin 500 mg three times daily.
- 2 weeks ago, still coughing, given clarithromycin. Body mass index 52. Chest X-ray arranged, and a follow-up appointment.

Current medication

- Just completed course of clarithromycin

Other clinical details

- 3 months ago – cholesterol 5.0, fasting glucose 5.3, creatinine 96 e GFR 70.
- Full blood count normal.
- Chest X-ray, 10 days ago.
- 'Upper lobe venous diversion, and increased cardiac diameter in keeping with left ventricular failure. No other abnormalities seen.'

<table>
<tr><td colspan="2">CSA Case Marking Sheet:
Case name: Jason Brown [Case 3]</td></tr>
<tr><td colspan="2">Focus for the case: Break news of heart failure, and work in collaboration with the patient to arrange appropriate investigation, pharmacological and non-pharmacological treatment</td></tr>
<tr><td>Data-gathering, technical and assessment skills</td><td>Obtains appropriate history, risk factors and abnormal investigation findings</td></tr>
<tr><td>Positive descriptors:
• Confirms that the history is in keeping with the report of the chest X-ray indicating left ventricular failure
• Recognises that risk factors include his body mass index and possibly his family history
• History ascertains that there is no suggestion of angina
• History explores diet and lifestyle
• Appropriate and well-conducted examination</td><td>Negative descriptors:
• Lacking in confidence in making a positive diagnosis, failure to interpret the data correctly
• Disorganised in arranging data to ascertain all risk factors
• Does not perform appropriately targeted or proficient examination
• Does not enquire regarding diet and lifestyle</td></tr>
<tr><td>Clinical Management skills</td><td>Arranges appropriate investigation and management of heart failure</td></tr>
<tr><td>Positive descriptors:
• Having recognised the presentation of heart failure to communicate this diagnosis effectively
• Initiate appropriate investigations that are likely to include ECG, FBC and repeat U&E monitoring (with treatment)
• Pro-brain natriuretic peptide and/or echocardiogram
• Commences appropriate management for heart failure. ACE inhibitor, and diuretic are likely to be commenced</td><td>Negative descriptors:
• Inadequate explanation of the diagnosis
• Does not undertake appropriate investigations
• Adequate or appropriate treatment not initiated
• Lacks confidence in monitoring treatment
• Interval and follow-up not specified, or inappropriate</td></tr>
</table>

Interpersonal skills	Is able to break bad news sensitively, and work in partnership with the patient
Positive descriptors: • Empathic manner while breaking bad news • Works in partnership with the patient to engage them positively in treatment • Able to convey seriousness of the condition without generating distress or unnecessary alarm • Approaches the problem positively to encourage patient in health promotion • Sensitive to the patient's feelings • Understands the impact on the patient's life of the new diagnosis • Is non-judgemental regarding weight and lifestyle	**Negative descriptors:** • Candidate does not appear comfortable breaking bad news leading to reduced quality consultation • Candidate not able to work in good partnership with the patient • Fails to understand the impact of the diagnosis on the patient • Approaches the problem narrowly failing to engage the patient in health promotion regarding their risk factors • Does not appear sympathetic to difficulties regarding weight management

Name of the 'Patient':	**Jason Brown** [Case 3]
Curriculum Clinical Statement	3.12 Cardiovascular health

This case is testing the candidate's ability to

- Show an understanding of the symptoms, signs and investigations for chronic heart failure
- Break the news of a potentially serious chronic condition to the patient in a sympathetic and effective manner
- Use the consultation to work towards empowering the patient and effective health promotion
- Commence appropriate treatment for heart failure, and show an understanding of an appropriate management plan for this condition
- Manage appropriately including pharmacological and lifestyle interventions.

Learning resources

Management of chronic heart failure – http://www.guidelines.co.uk/cardiovascular_nice_chronic_heart#.VE_l8DSsXXo.

Also, resources for breaking bad news and motivational interviewing are available.

General resources on communication skills are many and varied, with a range of consultation models.

Case 4

Name of 'Patient': Ian Marsden
Gender: Male
Age: 58

Background

- You run your own family building business
- you are married with two grown-up children

Opening statement

'I've been a bit of an idiot; I've really done something to my right leg doctor'

Information to give

2 weeks ago you were fooling around with your son in the gym – you keep fit and were a bit of a gymnast in your youth – you were demonstrating to your son how to do a backwards flip/hand-spring, you landed badly in a dip in the floor mat, and you felt something 'twang' in the back of your right leg.

- You weren't warmed up and you've not been to gym for years now – you've had too much work.
- It's been painful, so you've been taking some pain killers – Nurofen.
- You iced it.
- You did notice some bruising around the bottom of your ankle, but this has gone.

The CSA Exam: Maximizing your Success, First Edition. Rachel Roberts.

Companion Website: www.wiley.com\go\Roberts\CSAExam

- This happened at a weekend on a Saturday and, with all the adverts on the buses about not going to A&E 'unless you are dying', and because you felt such 'an idiot', you really didn't think you should … and within a few days the pain was settling, although it has remained tender and a bit swollen above and behind your ankle.
- The reason you have come now is that you have been busy on a job and are going on a holiday to Majorca the day after tomorrow … you wonder if there are some stronger pills you can take, so you will be more comfortable when you go.
- You used to play a bit of football – if asked you are right footed.

If specifically asked what you do/or about work/ how it has been affecting you

- You've been able to carry on at work and have done so, as you had a job to finish for a pushy client.
- You couldn't get an appointment with the doctor sooner.
- You have found difficulty up and down ladders and so have delegated this work.
- You have been having difficulty standing on tip toe, for example on the affected leg reaching up for things.
- You are right footed, or were when you played centre forward for the Camden Rovers FC.

If asked about general health:

- You are otherwise well, apart from a recent flare of epididymitis (which relapses occasionally following vasectomy 6 years ago), but this is now settled after the course of antibiotics the doctor gave you last time.

If asked about insurance:

- You have travel insurance taken out when you booked the holiday 3 months ago.
- You do not have private medical insurance.
- If advised to let your insurer know, ask 'why?'

Only if specifically asked

- No swelling behind knee (never had a 'Bakers Cyst' if asked about this).
- The calf has not been hot red or tender, you have no history of blood clots or DVT and no family history of such things.

You do not smoke and drink at weekends a couple of pints on average.

You will gladly accept 'some stronger pills' and coming back after your holiday, if doctor suggests this course of action.

Past medical history

- Appendicectomy 1998
- Vasectomy 2006
- Relapsing epididymitis 6 years ago – occasional course of ciprofloxacin
- No STDs
- Medication – recent course ciprofloxacin finished 4 weeks ago.

A knowledgeable doctor might ask if you have recently taken a specific type of antibiotic 'ciprofloxacin' – to which the answer is 'Yes, I finished a course about 1 month ago'

Questions to ask the doctor, if appropriate

- You are slightly resistant to going to A&E or any other urgent referral or investigation the doctor might suggest (US or X-ray) … 'Can it wait till after my 2-week holiday?'
- But you will go if doctor explains why … as you could have a complete rupture of Achilles tendon which may require you to be put into a cast or have a repair in order that you can walk normally and get back to normal working activities.
- If told how long you may have to be off work, you will be concerned to hear that this could be a few months and that you may require an operation and physiotherapy, as you have orders/jobs in hand – you will need to let your brother and son and clients know – it's a family business.
- 'Can I go on holiday … my wife's going to be livid … '
- The doctor may offer to phone orthopaedic team to arrange a clinic appointment in the next few days – you will respond positively to this – anything rather than sit around in A&E for hours!
- A good candidate might add something about the possibility of him needing DVT prophylaxis if hospital put him in plaster should this be added? – this hospital wil probably advise about this – but patient may need help from practice with prescription and showing hime how to do injections if necessary?
- You will accept routine referral for after your holiday if this is negotiated.
- If the doctor asks to examine you – 'Ok, what are you going to do?'
- If the candidate asks you to stand on tip toe, you can say: 'I tried that the other day and the funny thing was I couldn't do it'. If the candidate persists in wanting to examine you, try to perform a tip toe on your right leg but struggle.
- If the doctor asks about antibiotics – 'Why are you asking?', as it seems a bit nosy.

- If the doctor says this antibiotic has been linked to tendon inflammation and damage, act a bit surprised, but then say – 'Come to think of it, I did read about that on the leaflet a while back'

Behaviour/demeanour/body language

Chirpy and cheerful – but slightly embarrassed.
You want to work in partnership with the doctor.
You are not keen to go and wait in A&E, but will do so, if the reasons are explained.
Worried you may have to cancel your holiday next week.

Issues for preparation of the case

- Instructions to the 'Examiner':

The candidate should inspect and palpate – with permission – the right lower leg comparing with the unaffected side in either a prone position or kneeling on the patients chair examining affected/unaffected side alternately. If performed adequately, the examiner may verbally offer the information that –

'There is some boggy tender swelling in the lower right calf and a defect felt in the right Achilles tendon'

While inspecting, and with the permission of the patient, the candidate may ask, advise or demonstrate intent that they are gently going to squeeze the calf on the affected side (they may ask to do both sides). If this intent is demonstrated, the examiner may give the card below – or give the findings verbally.

Examination Card

When the right calf is squeezed, the foot does *not* plantar flex.

Materials for the doctor [displayed on the iPad in the CSA]

Case notes for the patient

Name:	Ian Marsden
Age:	45
Address:	15 Hampton Road

Social and family history

- Married
- 2 grown-up children

Past medical history

- Vasectomy 2003
- Appendicectomy 1999
- Recurrent epididymitis.

Current medication

- Recurrent epididymitis – repeat ciprofloxacin 500 bd for 2 weeks
- Diclofenac 50 mg tds for 2 weeks

Other clinical details

- Last consultation – 6 weeks ago

CSA Case Marking Sheet: Case name: Ian Marsden [Case 4]	
Focus for the case – Appropriate history taking examination and generation of an appropriate management plan. Social conflict/dilemma – holiday pending	
Data-gathering, technical and assessment skills	Solicits a history of tendon rupture and performs a competent physical examination
Positive descriptors: • Elicits symptoms of tendon rupture • Recognises the classic symptom a twang/snap in the back of the lower leg • Places symptoms in social context of work, delay in diagnosis and holiday • Asks about past medical history, medication treatment, e.g. quinolones • Excludes other possible causes • Adequate examination of the lower leg solicits Simmons/Thompsons test	**Negative descriptors:** • Does not recognise the classic history • Attributes pain to other cause • Does not solicit relevant social history work and holiday • Does not gather relevant past medical history and medication • Does not perform a competent examination
Clinical Management skills	Makes the diagnosis of tendon rupture and responds appropriately to the delay. Negotiates a management plan acceptable to the patient. Manages the interface between primary and secondary care

Positive descriptors: • Advises patient of probable diagnosis and potential impact of tendon rupture on mobility/function • Aware of likely management options conservative/repair • Works within limits of competence recommends and arranges further prompt investigation reference to A&E/urgent orthopaedics before holiday to help management decision, e.g. offers to discuss with secondary care • Suggests alternative treatment to quinolones for future bouts of epididymitis • Asks about holiday insurance. Suggests patient contacts travel insurers to advise them of this injury as a material fact	**Negative descriptors:** • Does not recognised the presentation and the dilemma for the patient and the doctor • Unaware of management options does not offer to arrange or recommend further assessment • Shows no resistance to patients desire to go on holiday the day after tomorrow without investigating further • Unaware of side effect of quinolones • Does not safety-net, e.g. fails to recommend contacting insurers
Interpersonal skills	Is sympathetic to the patient's self-recrimination and social situation and works in partnership to achieve an agreed outcome
Positive descriptors: • Active listening acknowledges impact short and long terms • Works around patient resistance • Willing to be flexible in approach, e.g. considers facilitated offers to liaise secondary care or encourages A&E/emergency unit attendance	**Negative descriptors:** • Dismissive of symptoms • Collusive with pts desire not to 'be a nuisance' • Inflexible in approach

Name of the patient:	**Ian Marsden** [Case 4]
Curriculum Clinical Statement	3.20 Care of people with Musculoskeletal Problems

This case is testing the candidate's ability to

- Diagnose a ruptured Achilles tendon from history and appropriately attempted examination
- Recognise the level of urgency with which this should be treated
- Navigate the patient to an appropriate level of care
- Be willing to negotiate with the patient and liaise with secondary care to achieve an appropriate management plan
- Use time and resources appropriately in a manner that demonstrates and prioritises management appreciation of potential for loss of function impact on employment and future mobility
- Recognise the potential impact on his forthcoming holiday and dealing with uncertainty around this. Safety-net appropriately.

Learning resources

There is an excellent account of Achilles tendon rupture presentations and management options on 'Patient.co.uk'.

Case 5

Name of 'Patient':	**Gavin South**
Gender:	Male
Age:	38
BMI:	33

Background

- You have had diarrhoea since you went on holiday 6 weeks ago to Egypt.
- You are employed as a Chef, catering for a corporate bank in the City of London, preparing lunches and dinners for corporate clients. It is a high-pressure work.
- You live with your long-term partner, Alistair, who is a fashion designer.
- You have been seeing each other for 10 years.
- You love travelling.
- You enjoy the gay lifestyle, you are not promiscuous, but you have your doubts about Alistair sometimes. You both have regular HIV tests and have always tested negative. The most recent test was 2 weeks ago after coming back from holiday – it was negative.
- Your elderly parents live 'up north'. Your Mum has colitis which she developed in her 20s. Dad is well, fit as an ox. You see them occasionally but are not in touch as much as you would like.
- You have a sister, Sheila, who lives in Sydney, Australia, and with whom you keep in touch. You saw her last year at Christmas.

Opening statement

'I've had really bad diarrhoea, doctor'

The CSA Exam: Maximizing your Success, First Edition. Rachel Roberts.

Companion Website: www.wiley.com\go\Roberts\CSAExam

Information to give, if asked specifically by the doctor

- When asked what the problem is – you've been going to the toilet all the time since you came back from Egypt – up to 6 times a day.
- Loose watery stool.
- Occasional blood and mucus – but this is getting less.
- Possibly a bit feverish when you came back from holiday, but it's settled, just some gripes still now and again.
- You've had occasional episodes of traveller's diarrhoea in the past – but nothing that has gone on like this. It stopped and started a bit, but you've been going to work although you think perhaps you should not have.
- You are really worried, as it's been going on a bit.
- Your boss said you had to see the doctor.
- Your partner is really worried too.
- Your mum has ulcerative colitis and has regular bowel checks and takes mesalazine – or something. She had to have a colostomy about 10 years ago because she had cancerous changes.
- If asked if you are gay? – 'Well yeah' (as if it's fairly obvious but not taking offence).
- You and your partner have recently gone for a full sexual health screen together. You are HIV negative,
- You had an appendicectomy when you were 25 – they did it all by telescope – no complications.
- You don't smoke.
- You drink vodka more than you should – you reckon honestly you drink about 30–40 units a week (40 if you have a heavy week clubbing). The diarrhoea has been worse after drinking last weekend.
- You have taken a bit of cocaine in the distant past – but not for the last 10 years.
- No other recent traumas or life events.
- Slight weight loss, no severe sweats or palpitations.

Questions to ask the doctor, if appropriate

If the doctor proposes blood tests

- You should agree, but ask what for and why?
- Do you think this could be HIV related? (If doctor hasn't covered this or reassured you about it)

If the doctor proposes a stool test

- Ask how you do this? – the doctor may say something like – if you ask at reception they will give you a kit and advice leaflet.

If asked your ideas about what you think might be going on –

- You thought it might be just something persisting after your holiday.

If asked what you thought might happen today –

- You thought you might need some antibiotics and be able to go back to work.

If doctor proposes further tests and coming back

- Isn't there something you can do for me today … ?
- Can you give me something to stop me going?

If the doctor doesn't advise about work

Ask 'Am I Ok to go back to work?'

If the doctor says yes, say 'great I was hoping you'd say that'.
If the doctor says no, say 'Oh dear, why?'

The doctor should explain that because you handle food and have been travelling, it is important to make sure that your motions are clear of any infection – and that public health may need to be involved – You should be advised to tell your line manager you are waiting for results.

If doctor explains this, say you will need a certificate. The doctor should advise a self-certificate – If so, ask how that works. You haven't been off sick for years.

Another possibility here is inflammatory bowel disease. You will need to wait for the results of blood tests and consider further investigation.

Behaviour/demeanour/body language

Slightly embarrassed and anxious

Issues for Preparation of the case

Physical Examination

- *Pulse blood pressure and temperature are normal.*
- The doctor should examine your abdomen which is generally a bit tender. There is no lymphadenopathy.
- Rectal examination should be offered – including a chaperone, which you decline.
- The examiner will intervene to advise the examination is 'normal'.

Materials for the doctor [displayed on the iPad in the CSA]

Case notes for the patient

Name:	Gavin South
Age:	38
Address:	69 Garston Road

Social and family history

- Lives with partner
- Family history – Mother Colitis – colostomy

Past medical history

- Laparoscopic appendicectomy 1999

Current medication

- Nil
- Allergies nil

Other clinical details

- Travel immunisations
- Updated 3 months ago including Hep A Typhoid
- Non-smoker

CSA Case Marking Sheet: Case name: Gavin South [Case 5]	
Focus for the case: Ascertain social and occupational information in relation to diarrhoea, and reach an appropriate differential diagnosis. Good communication skills, respecting equality and diversity.	
Data-gathering, technical and assessment skills	Thorough assessment including medical psychological and social factors
Positive descriptors: • Takes full history covering medical and psychosocial factors including occupation, travel immunisations • Assesses lifestyle factors appropriately, e.g. drugs, alcohol, smoking, safe sex • Asks about duration and nature of physical symptoms tiredness, frequency, looseness, blood, mucus, weight loss covers red flags • Offers appropriate examination • Attention to personal hygiene, e.g. hand washing/cleansing after examination	**Negative descriptors:** • Omits important aspects of history • Does not respond to worries about partner • Makes assumptions about psycho-social causation • Does not offer examination • Does not examine for lymphadenopathy • Does not offer rectal examination • No attention to personal hygiene after examination if offered (this is a case of potentially infectious diarrhoea)
Clinical Management skills	Management plan for in line with current best practice and agreeable to the patient

Positive descriptors: • Makes a differential diagnosis of possible traveller's or inflammatory bowel disease. Considers alternative diagnoses such as Inflammatory Bowel Disease, seroconversion illness, alcohol excess • Gives advice about work and need for him to liaise with occupational health • Covers certification • Offers appropriate tests – fbc, esr crp coeliac screen • Stool test • Proposes appropriate intervention waiting for stool sample before return to work • Suggest referral if symptoms aren't settling • Encourages reduction of alcohol consumption	**Negative descriptors:** • Fails to offer investigation • Poor tolerance of uncertainty • Doesn't cover occupational factors • Unaware of self-certification procedure • Does not accommodate worry about seroconversion illness
Interpersonal skills	Demonstrate a professional and non-judgemental approach respecting equality and diversity
Positive descriptors: • Matter-of-fact, non-judgemental approach • Good rapport • Sensitive to worries about partner • Able to encourage lifestyle approach realistically tailored to patient	**Negative descriptors:** • Judgemental response • Proscriptive approach • Unsympathetic about impact on life and work • Does not address worry in case of inflammatory bowel diagnosis

Name of the 'Patient': **Gavin South** [Case 5]
Curriculum Clinical Statement: Digestive health

This case is testing the candidate's ability to

- Take a full history and offer appropriate examination and tests investigation as appropriate
- Manage public health and occupational factors in partnership with the patient
- Be able to manage primary contact with patients who have a digestive problem
- Understand the epidemiology of digestive problems as they present in primary care and their often complex aetiology
- Know how to interpret common symptoms in general practice, including weight loss, rectal bleeding, diarrhoea
- Demonstrate a systematic approach to investigating common digestive symptoms, taking into account the prevalence of these symptoms in primary care
- Understand that digestive symptoms are frequently linked to psycho-social factors and empathise with individuals who are psychologically distressed
- Be sensitive to context e.g. a gayman worried about seroconversion illness
- Explore gastrointestinal symptoms and psychological and social factors using an integrated approach
- Understand the range of gastrointestinal problems associated with alcohol and drug usage.

Learning resources

http://www.patient.co.uk/doctor/chronic-diarrhoea-in-adults.

Case 6

Name of 'Patient': **Louise Bradley**
Gender: Female
Age: 61

Background

- Lives with husband
- Two daughters, grown up, left home. Both live locally and are very supportive

Opening statement

'I am not sure if I should be troubling you with this, but 2 weeks ago I had a slight brown discharge'

Information to give

If asked where from? It was from the front. This has not happened to you since your last period about 10 years ago.

Information to give, if asked specifically by the doctor

- There has been no bleeding. This was light brown discharge which lasted about 3 days. You had no pain, soreness or itching.
- *If asked directly* – you were on tamoxifen for 5 years after the breast operation and stopped it about 18 months ago.
- *If asked directly* – you did ask your daughters to see their GPs because of the family history of breast cancer and they are being followed up.

The CSA Exam: Maximizing your Success, First Edition. Rachel Roberts.

Companion Website: www.wiley.com\go\Roberts\CSAExam

- *If asked directly* – you have taken HRT for your menopause symptoms from the age of 50–54 and were asked to stop it when you were diagnosed with breast cancer.
- You stopped smoking when you were diagnosed with breast cancer.
- Alcohol socially, just at weekends – two glasses of wine shared with your husband.
- Patients ideas, concerns and expectations:

  I – you think it may be related to sex you had 3 weeks ago,

  C – you are concerned in case this recurs – you have no idea what is causing it.

  E – you want a cream or medication to prevent it recurring.

Past medical history

- Age 23 – appendicectomy
- Age 54 – breast cancer
- Age 54 – lumpectomy left breast.
- Age 55 – hypertension.

Your last smear test was 6 years ago – Normal

Medication

- Amlodipine 5 mg daily

Family history

Father died in his late 70s due to heart problems. Mother still alive, has high blood pressure and had breast cancer in her late 50s.

Expect the doctor to ask to examine you

- The doctor should ask to do an intimate examination of the vulva, the vagina and the cervix. The 'Examiner' or 'Patient' will interrupt to say that all is 'normal'.
- The doctor may suggest repeating a smear test – say you will see the nurse.

Questions to ask the doctor, if appropriate

- Is there anything I can take to prevent this happening again?
- If the Dr mentions that there could be a problem with the lining of your womb – ask what exactly does that mean?

- If the Dr does not mention the word 'cancer', ask if this could be serious?
- If the Dr mentions the word 'cancer' – then you will look concerned and ask what happens next?
- You will also ask specifically what treatment will be needed if this is womb cancer?
- Also ask if this will need regular follow-up like the breast cancer for many years?

Behaviour/demeanour/body language

Concerned, co-operative but a little shy initially, and willing to accept doctor's management of hospital referral.

Issues for Preparation of the case

- Instructions to the person playing the 'Examiner':

If the candidate offers to examine the patient, please interrupt and say 'normal'.

If only two people are doing the role-play, the 'Patient' will say 'normal'.

Materials for the doctor [displayed on the iPad in the CSA]

Case notes for the patient:

Name: Louise Bradley
Age: 61
Address: 7 Manor Road

Social and family history

- Lives with husband.

Past medical history

- Age 23 – appendicectomy
- Age 54 – breast cancer
- Age 54 – lumpectomy left breast.
- Age 55 – hypertension.

Current medication

- Amlodipine 5 mg daily

Previous consultations

- 1 month ago

New patient check with your nurse – BP 134/82; p 73; urinalysis – NAD
BMI: 26

CSA Case Marking Sheet: Case name: Louise Bradley [Case 6]	
Focus for the case: The candidate's ability to manage a patient with PMB and additional risk factors. Arranging suitable investigation and management	
Data-gathering, technical and assessment skills	Gathers focused history and examination to confirm PMB and additional risk factors
Positive descriptors: • Gathers information to confirm degree duration of PMB • Focused history, consider risk factors for PMB – tamoxifen • Explores impact on her and family • Examination is offered • Good candidate picks up family history of breast cancer	**Negative descriptors:** • Disorganised gathering of data • Fails to identify risk factor of tamoxifen • Focuses narrowly on the problem and does not identify family history of breast cancer • Examination not offered
Clinical Management skills	Shows awareness of correct management of PMB and health promotion (smear and family breast screening)
Positive descriptors: • Explains diagnoses and probability of uterine cancer • Explains possible link with tamoxifen • Arranges smear test • Explains and arranges 2-week-wait referral to gynaecology • Suggests daughters have breast screening • Follow-up after investigations and treatment completed in hospital	**Negative descriptors:** • Candidate does not appear to reach appropriate diagnoses • Management includes swab and reassurance • Fails to explain potential cancer • Failure to encourage smear test • Failure to refer 2-week wait • Fails to suggest daughters' breast screening • No follow-up arrangements

Case 6

Interpersonal skills	Facilitates patient's contribution and explains medical management, taking account patient's knowledge and expectations
Positive descriptors: • Active listening, and appropriately responds to the patient's concerns … • Provides relevant explanation of possible effect of tamoxifen • Maintains warmth, sympathy and understanding, while explaining possibility of uterine cancer • Takes into consideration the impact on her and her family	**Negative descriptors:** • Poor active listening skills • Causes unnecessary anxiety in the patient, while explaining 2-week wait and potential uterine cancer • Explanations of potential causes such as tamoxifen not discussed • Manner lacks warmth and understanding of the impact on her and the family

Name of 'Patient':	**Louise Bradley** [Case 6]
Curriculum Clinical Statements:	3.06 Women's Health 3.01 Healthy people: promoting health and preventing disease

This case is testing the candidate's ability to

- Confirm history of postmenopausal bleeding and family history of breast cancer
- Offer examination and cervical smear
- Develop a safe management plan
- Suggest screening for daughters
- Communicate sensitively the 2-week-wait referral to gynaecology.

Learning resources

http://www.patient.co.uk/doctor/postmenopausal-bleeding.
http://www.sign.ac.uk/guidelines/fulltext/61/section3.html.
http://www.patient.co.uk/doctor/breast-cancer-pro.

Case 7

Name of 'Patient': Jenny Stanley
Gender: Female
Age: 39

Background

- Works as machine operator in Bank of England printing works
- Married to Jack, a mechanic
- Two children – Brian age 10 and Louise age 12 – both well

Opening statement

'My husband is really starting to moan at me, can you do anything to help me?'

Information to give

- You've always had a tendency to snore, but in the last few weeks your husband has had to sleep in a separate room because of the disturbance.
- You have read in the newspaper that there may be some laser treatment available to stop this snoring noise.
- You have started to feel very self-conscious about this.
- You already don't feel very attractive, as you feel you are overweight, but this has now reduced your confidence even more.
- You have not had any other symptoms from your nose. In the daytime, you can breathe perfectly well.
- You have not had any past operations on your nose or your ears and do not suffer from hay fever or any other allergies.
- You do not smoke and you drink about four glasses of wine a week.

The CSA Exam: Maximizing your Success, First Edition. Rachel Roberts.

Companion Website: www.wiley.com\go\Roberts\CSAExam

Information to give, if asked specifically by the doctor

- You are feeling increasingly tired and can fall asleep very easily. There have been a few incidents recently at work of nodding off at the desk, and your supervisor is rather unhappy about your performance in recent weeks because of this.
- You do drive a car but have had no accidents or problems with falling asleep at the wheel.
- You are around 5 ft 2 in. (157 cm) and your weight is 15 1/2 stone (98 kg); this is an increase in 1 1/2 stone in the last year.
- You do not exercise; sometimes you walk to the shops, but nothing other than this. You certainly feel too tired now to take up any more vigorous exercise at the moment.
- You do try to eat a balanced diet, and to give the same to your children. Your portions are a little above ideal, and you do tend to have a liking for ice cream everyday for pudding.
- You do not feel depressed, and have no other symptoms of any kind.
- You have always got on well with your husband. You have a good relationship, but the snoring is spoiling this at present.
- You had a health check with the nurse 2 months ago, she took your blood pressure, weight and some blood tests. She said you needed to lose weight, and your cholesterol was not perfect, but that everything else was 'ok'.

Questions to ask the doctor, if appropriate

- 'So would this Laser treatment, I've read about, stop me snoring?'
- If the Dr offers to refer for this, ask if it will be available on the NHS.
- If the doctor suggests a sleep apnoea questionnaire, agree, but sound concerned and not very happy, if the doctor suggests you would wear a mask at night.
- If the doctor suggests you may not be able to drive because of falling asleep, become very worried – how will you get the children to school and back?

Behaviour/demeanour/body language

Rather shy and keen to get help from the doctor. No sign of appearing depressed.

Issues for preparation of the case

- Instructions to the person playing the 'Examiner':

  If the candidate offers to examine the patient, after the examination has been completed, please offer the card, or give the findings verbally appropriate to the examination undertaken.

  If only two people are doing the role-play, the 'Patient' will give the card, or give the findings verbally appropriate to the examination undertaken.

Examination Card

BMI 39.5

BP 140/83

Examination of ears, nose and throat – redundant tissue folds in oropharynx, otherwise normal.

Materials for the doctor [displayed on the iPad in the CSA]

Case notes for the patient:

Name:	Jenny Stanley
Age:	39
Address:	42 Thornhill Road

Social and family history

- Married to Jack
- Two children – Brian, age 10 and Louise age 12 – normal deliveries
- Ex-smoker, stopped 5 years ago

Past medical history

None

Current medication

None

Other clinical details

6 weeks ago saw the nurse

- BMI 39.5
- Blood pressure 135/75
- Cholesterol 5.5, HDL 1.0, LDL 3.5, triglycerides 1.7
- Fasting glucose 5.8
- Thyroid function normal

CSA Case Marking Sheet: Case name: Jenny Stanley [Case 7]	
Focus: Identifying that this person may be suffering from obstructive sleep apnoea, and arranging appropriate assessment. Addressing the psychological and social impact	
Data-gathering, technical and assessment skills	Explores the problem systematically, including the physical, social and psychological issues
Positive descriptors: • Identifies history suggestive of sleep apnoea, as well as snoring • Identifies the degree of somnolence and assess risks of this, e.g. driving • Identifies the impact on the patient's confidence and relationship • Identifies the patient's expectations • Enquires regarding any symptoms of depression	**Negative descriptors:** • Tackles snoring directly, without assessing for wider issues of sleep apnoea • Does not assess for risks of somnolence • Does not assess impact on confidence or relationship • Does not assess for depression • Does not explore patient expectations
Clinical Management skills	Shows a comprehensive approach, targeting appropriate investigation, lifestyle and psychological issues
Positive descriptors: • Recommends assessment which is likely to include an Epworth questionnaire to assess sleepiness and then assessment for sleep study • Is aware of referral processes and how to access assessment • Recommends lifestyle change in addition to impact of reducing BMI • Explains to the patient the assessment and likely treatment for sleep apnoea – CPAP	**Negative descriptors:** • ENT referral or agreement to assess for laser treatment of palate a negative indicator • Unaware of the ability to access sleep studies, and likely management • Does not manage the lifestyle factors • Addresses patient's problem narrowly

Interpersonal skills	Empathy and sensitivity is shown to the patient's concerns, with ability to engage and empower the patient
Positive descriptors: • Sympathetic manner, allowing patient to outline her lack of confidence • Good active listening • Able to negotiate appropriate assessment, and possibly unappealing treatment, without alienating the patient • Able to empower the patient to make some changes	**Negative descriptors:** • Inappropriately agrees to the patient's requests, as unable to adequately negotiate • Does not respond to patient concerns • Doctor-centred approach • Does not manage to negotiate a shared management of the problem

Name of the 'Patient': **Jenny Stanley** [Case 7]
Curriculum Clinical Statement: 3.15 Care of people who have ENT, oral and facial problems

This case is testing the candidate's ability to

- Identify a likely history of sleep apnoea, with its associated symptoms and risks, e.g. driving
- Arrange appropriate assessment for sleep apnoea, including an explanation of likely treatments
- Manage the problem holistically, including the effect on the patient's life, and including lifestyle interventions.

Learning resources

https://www.brit-thoracic.org.uk/clinical-information/sleep-apnoea.
http://www.blf.org.uk/Page/Obstructive-sleep-apnoea-OSA-health-information.

Case 8

Name of 'Patient':	**Harry Evans**
Gender:	Male
Age:	62

Background

- Works as an architect, in a firm in the local town
- Lives with wife who is now retired
- Two grown-up children who live some distance away

Opening statement

'I noticed all these bruises yesterday, doctor, and I don't remember doing anything to cause them'

Information to give

- You have never noticed unusual bruising before, and you haven't been doing any unusual activities lately.
- You can't think of any particular reason why these should have suddenly come up.
- You feel fine, a little more tired recently, but otherwise fine.
- You are eating well, doing all your normal activities, sleeping well and have had no temperature or any other symptoms.
- You are not bleeding from anywhere.
- You have never heard of anyone else getting this problem and have no idea what may have caused it.

The CSA Exam: Maximizing your Success, First Edition. Rachel Roberts.

Companion Website: www.wiley.com\go\Roberts\CSAExam

- You don't drink more than a glass of wine a week and you do not smoke.
- You have been working in the same firm of architects for many years, and there are no real changes or new stresses at work. You do work hard and felt that may have been the reason of you being a little tired recently.
- Your mood is fine and you have no real worries in your home life.
- You may be asked if you are breathless, having fevers, a headache or other symptoms – particularly to check for anaemia. You do not have any other symptoms.

Information to give, if asked specifically by the doctor:

- You are taking warfarin for your irregular heart beat. You are extremely careful to stick to the doses advised, and don't think you have made any mistakes with your doses.
- Your next blood test is due in 2 weeks.
- You do not take any other medication but if specifically prompted about any over-the-counter medication, you can mention that you bought some herbal remedy for tiredness which you started last week.
- You have not suffered any blows or physical trauma of any kind.
- Atrial fibrillation diagnosed 3 years ago on warfarin.
- Myelofibrosis – diagnosed 2 years ago. You had a series of blood tests and scan.
- You were told that the situation didn't require any current treatment 2 years ago, and you have not received any follow-up appointment or blood test since

Questions to ask the doctor, if appropriate

- 'Is this dangerous doctor?'
- 'Will these go away on their own?'
- If offered admission, ask 'You must be really worried doctor, why is it necessary?'

Behaviour/demeanour/body language

Calm, co-operative and rather puzzled. If admission is suggested, become anxious.

Expect the doctor to ask to examine you

Issues for Preparation of the case:
Instructions to the person playing the 'Examiner':

After examination has been completed, please offer the card below – Or give the findings verbally appropriate to the examination undertaken.
If only two people are doing the role-play, the 'Patient' will give the card – Or give the findings verbally appropriate to the examination undertaken.

Examination Card

Looks well, temperature 36.6 °C. No apparent clinical anaemia.
Multiple bruises on arms, legs and trunk, largest is up to 5 cm, others are around 1 or 2 cm.
Pulse 72 atrial fibrillation, blood pressure 120/75.
No lymph nodes palpable in any area.
No hepatomegaly, but significant splenomegaly.

Materials for the doctor [displayed on the iPad in the CSA]

Case notes for the patient:

Name:	Harry Evans
Age:	62
Address:	14 Stanton Drive

Social and family history

- Architect in a local firm

Past medical history

- Atrial fibrillation diagnosed 3 years ago.
- Myelofibrosis – diagnosed 2 years ago. Outpatient letter about the myelofibrosis 2 years ago. Detailing no medication needed at that point, but for regular review.
- No outpatient letters since.

Current medication

- Warfarin 3 mg
- Bisoprolol 5 mg
- Last INR 3 weeks ago 2.2

CSA Case Marking Sheet: **Case name: Harry Evans [Case 8]**	
Focus for the case: Recognise abnormal bruising, consider appropriate differential diagnoses as to the cause and act with appropriate urgency to manage this case	
Data-gathering, technical and assessment skills	Elucidate history of spontaneous bruising and assess potential causes
Positive descriptors: • History elucidates very short history of spontaneous bruising • Focused history to ascertain tiredness , but absence of any other systemic symptoms • Explores possible links to warfarin or to history of myelofibrosis • Examination is focused to include skin, temperature, lymph node areas, liver and spleen • Good candidate picks up over-the-counter herbal remedy	**Negative descriptors:** • Disorganised gathering of data which does not appear guided by probabilities of disease • Focuses narrowly on the problem, for example only concentrating on warfarin with no exploration of any other potential symptoms or causes • Examination does not include the relevant focused elements or is conducted with poor technique
Clinical Management skills	Develop a management plan which is safe and includes appropriate urgency
Positive descriptors: • Recognises the significance of the symptoms, and the potential underlying causes of either INR derangement or complications of myelofibrosis • Safe management of urgency of situation, to include a same-day blood test and may withhold next-day warfarin until result known • Management includes considering possible links with myelofibrosis, so reinstates appropriate opinion. This is with appropriate urgency	**Negative descriptors:** • Candidate does not appear to reach appropriate differential diagnoses • Management is not conducted with appropriate urgency or safety • Follow-up arrangements regarding previous myelofibrosis is inadequate • Candidate does not make safe arrangements for INR and warfarin adjustment

Interpersonal skills	Communicate information regarding medical problems and risk effectively, while maintaining a calm interaction with the patient and good rapport
Positive descriptors: • Active listening, and appropriately responds to possibly urgent problem without alarming the patient • Provides relevant explanation of possible link of bruising to either medication interaction or underlying medical problem, in terms understandable to the patient • Maintains warmth and understanding while exploring the symptoms and possible causes	**Negative descriptors:** • Poor active listening skills • Causes unnecessary anxiety in the patient • Explanations of potential causes are not relevant or appropriate to the patient • Manner lacks warmth and understanding

Name of the 'Patient':	Harry Evans [Case 8]
Curriculum Clinical Statement:	3.03 – Care of acutely ill people

This case is testing the candidate's ability to

- Elucidate history of spontaneous bruising
- Identify potential causes from the information given to candidates and the patient history
- Perform a focused examination of bruising, haemopoetic and lymphatic system
- Generate a management plan which incorporates the most likely diagnoses with appropriate urgency
- Communicate information regarding medical problems and risk effectively, while maintaining a calm interaction with the patient.

Learning resources

http://www.patient.co.uk/doctor/oral-anticoagulants.
Guideline for the diagnosis and management of myelofibrosis.
http://onlinelibrary.wiley.com/doi/10.1111/j.1365-2141.2012.09179.x/pdf.

Case 9

Name of 'Patient': **Shona Baker**
Gender: Female
Age: 15 years, 7 months

Background

- You live with mum and younger brother, Tobias, who is 'a pain'
- Dad left when you were little – you don't have much to do with him
- you school nearby – "Beech Park"
- You want to leave after GCSEs and train to be a beautician
- Going steady with a boy in year above – mum has told you to 'be careful'

Opening statement

'My mum sent me. She thinks I ought to go on the pill'

Information to give

- Periods have been heavy painful and irregular since they started about 2 years ago.
- You have tried Nurofen which helps a bit.
- One of your mates came to see the nurse here a few weeks ago and said the nurse had advised her to go on the Pill – she said the nurse was really good but you couldn't get to see her today so have come to the doctor instead.

The CSA Exam: Maximizing your Success, First Edition. Rachel Roberts.

Companion Website: www.wiley.com\go\Roberts\CSAExam

Information to give, if asked specifically by the candidate

- You will be 16 in 5 months.
- You haven't missed any periods and you are due on in a few days.
- You started smoking a bit after school with mates, at most 5 a day.
- Alcohol occasionally at parties, your boyfriend drinks a bit more.
- No drugs.
- Mum couldn't come today because she is at work (flower shop).
- You are not fully sexually active – but you are in a relationship with a boy in the year above at school who is being 'a bit pushy'.
- If asked are you being forced into anything – 'No, not at all' – but you are worried about things going a bit further.
- You are not worried about any sexually transmitted diseases (STDs) – you had a big talk on STDs and chlamydia and all that at school.
- Your boyfriend hasn't ever tried to get you drunk.
- Your mum has said you ought to go on the pill. She had similar problem with periods, and she knows about the relationship and wants you to be careful.
- She has told you to make sure, if he tries it on, to use condoms which, to be honest, you already have done and you've played around a bit....
- 'You ain't gonna to tell my Mum, are you?' If doctor reassures you and tells you that everything is confidential, you are reassured.
- You have done a pregnancy test which was negative.
- If the doctor suggests that you make an appointment with mum, you are agreeable but can't I have something now – 'my period is due in a few days'.
- If the doctor asks whether you think you might be at risk of falling pregnant or similar ... you are a bit worried, and think your mum is too.
- A good doctor may try quite hard to suggest other methods – for example injection – refuse, you really hate needles. If offered information, you'll have a look.
- If doctor says it's a good idea to carry on using condoms as well – say 'yeah they told us that at school, especially if you change partners – but I ain't planning to!'
- You have never suffered with migraines or any type of headache – if doctor says migraine ask 'what do you mean?'– there is no family history of these.
- Likewise no history or family history of blood clots in legs or lungs if doctors says DVT or PE, ask 'what do you mean?'

Questions for the role-player to ask the doctor, if appropriate

- If doctor offers alternatives for period pain, you are happy to accept these, 'but is there anything else I could try?'
- 'When should I start taking this pill?'
- 'Are there any side effects … my mate said it can cause breast cancer?'
- 'Will these tablets help my skin?'
- 'Is it right that having sex under 16 is against the law?'
- 'Do I need to start having smears regularly?'

Behaviour/demeanour/body language

Cheerful, perhaps a bit older than your years, but not precocious. Sensible young person but not terribly forthcoming with answers. Not embarrassed, enjoys being a bit challenging.

Instructions to examiner

If the candidate wants to take BP, the 'Examiner' will intervene and disclose the information. If only two people are doing the role-play, the 'Patient' will give the BP result.

Examination Card

BP normal 121/79

Materials for the doctor [displayed on the iPad in the CSA]

Case notes for the patient:

Name:	Shona Baker
Age:	15
Address:	6, St Mungo's Court

Social and family history

- Lives with Mum and younger brother
- Attends Beech Park school

Past medical history

- None

Current medication

- Nil

Other clinical details

- No allergies
- Fully Immunised
- BCG and MMR HPV – up to date

CSA Case Marking Sheet: Case name: Shona Baker [Case 9]	
Focus for the case: Assessing risk of unplanned pregnancy and providing appropriate contraceptive advice	
Data-gathering, technical and assessment skills	Demonstrate ability to take an adequate sexual health history from a teenage girl and assess risk of unplanned pregnancy
Positive descriptors: • Establishes the reason for attendance • Takes menstrual history including dysmenorrhoea • Exclude possible pregnancy • Explore risk of unplanned pregnancy • Takes social history / school etc • Establishes young person at risk of pregnancy • Explores for risk taking behaviour, including alcohol and drugs • Excludes exploitation • Covers HPV vaccination • Asks about history of migraine, smoking, VTE • Takes blood pressure	**Negative descriptors:** • Fails to explore dysmenorrhoea • Fails to exclude possible pregnancy and risk of unplanned pregnancy • Does not establish social background • Does not ask about medical risk factors – migraine smoking, venous thromboembolism • Does not ask about risk-taking behaviours • Does not take BP • Reflexly prescribes ocp
Clinical Management skills	Offers appropriate and comprehensive contraceptive advice tailored to the young persons' preferences

Positive descriptors: • Adequately establishes competence of young person with respect to Fraser rules • Promotes LARC as method of choice • Safely prescribes ocp with appropriate advice on when to start • Safety-nets if no period or concerned in case of possible pregnancy, e.g. repeat test • Offers leaflet, advises to read prescribing information or speak to pharmacist • Offers advice about smoking • Covers cancer benefit/risk adequately • Offers advice about emergency contraception and missed pill and safe sex • Recommends follow-up with self and or other team members	**Negative descriptors:** • Prescribes inappropriately • Fails to assess risk of pregnancy and take a preventive approach • Fails to give opportunistic advice about, e.g. smoking, alcohol, sexual health • Fails to safety-net or promote other services including pharmacy/ practice nurse etc • Gives wrong advice about starting oc or fails to provide leaflets, etc. • Fails to safety-net re no period • Fails to offer follow-up
Interpersonal skills	Puts young person at ease and involves them in management decisions, maintains effective working relationship
Positive descriptors: • Establishes rapport and maintains professional approach • Covers any issue of confidentiality and puts patient at ease • Non-judgemental • Promotes involvement of parent in decision making and healthy choices	**Negative descriptors:** • Fails to form rapport while maintaining a professional and comprehensive approach • Refuses the OC, no offer of alternative professional help/provision of need • General approach likely to deter young person from seeking advice again

Name of the patient: Shona Baker [Case 9]
Curriculum Clinical Statement: 3.04 Care of Children and Young People

This case is testing the candidate's ability to

- Gain the trust of the patient
- Assess whether she is at any risk of harm/abuse
- Communicate information regarding contraceptive choices, maintaining an effective working relationship with the young person promoting appropriate access to health-care services
- (In the event that they have personal moral or religious objections to provision of such services) signpost the patient to alternative services in a non-judgemental manner.

Learning resources

http://www.fpa.org.uk/resources/downloads.
http://www.fsrh.org/pdfs/ceuGuidanceYoungPeople2010.pdf.

Case 10

Name of 'Patient':	**Amelia Kowalski**
Gender:	Female
Age:	35

Background

- Polish bar worker.
- You have lived in the United Kingdom last 10 years and are settled here.
- Your partner, Phil, is a local builder.
- Your children are at school locally.
- You work hard with long hours the last year or so.

Opening statement

'It's my nails doctor they are dreadful – I have taken a picture of them'

Information to give

- Work environment is hot, your feet and hands often get wet with bar slops towards end of shift and at times your feet now are becoming uncomfortable.
- You enjoy swimming – but your feet are getting embarrassing.
- Your partner doesn't like your feet, and your two children (Karen aged 4, Steve aged 5) are teasing you about it. None of them has any rashes.
- A doctor back home in Poland told you to use some paint which you have been using but are finding products expensive over the counter and they are not really working.
- You are so embarrassed that you keep your nails painted the whole time, but you have taken a picture of the worst-affected fingers and toes and 'here it is' on your phone/or you have printed it off for the doctor.

The CSA Exam: Maximizing your Success, First Edition. Rachel Roberts.

Companion Website: www.wiley.com\go\Roberts\CSAExam

- You suffer with migraine which has been much better since you started the propranolol a few months ago.
- Your fingers and toes nails are getting thicker, and they are hard to trim.
- Toes hurt when they press on the inside of a shoe which they do towards the end of your shift.
- You keep them painted all the time now because of the embarrassment. Your finger nails bother you most.
- You get some itching especially between the 4th and 5th toes.
- You daren't go swimming any more – you are worried about spreading it to other people.
- The nails worst affected are the big and little toes. Thick and crumbly, and getting deformed.
- The nails are damaging your socks.
- Sometimes, the skin around the nail gets red and swollen, but it is alright now.

Information to give, if asked specifically by the doctor

- Just lately your toes and fingers have been hurting a bit at the end of your bar shift.
- It is the ***fingertip*** and ***toe tip*** joints that hurt.
- You sometimes get some back ache from moving the barrels around.
- You have had some rash on your elbows for years which has been a bit flaky (you have a picture of this too). You remember it got better when you were pregnant.
- You think the rash on your elbows has got a bit worse since starting the propranolol.
- You may be getting some of it on the front of your knees too *(do not volunteer this).*
- If asked if there is a family history of skin conditions – your mother has a bad scaly condition but you do not know what it is.
- Your parents live in Warsaw and you see them at Christmas.
- If the doctor suggests taking a nail scraping, you agree to this, and are happy to come back, having removed your nail polish.
- You are not too bothered about elbows and knees at present but are happy to try a bit of treatment for this if recommended.
- You really do not want to stop the propranolol as it has really helped your migraines … but you will think about it if the rash gets worse.
- You are not diabetic no other health problems

Questions to ask the doctor, if appropriate

- Why are you asking about joint pain?
- What is causing it?
- Can I give it to other people?
- Why do I have to wait for the test results – my friend went to her GP and he just gave her some tablets?
- If doctor suggests referral, ask why and to whom?
- Can I carry on using the nail paints for the time being?
- Can I have a prescription for a few months – it's expensive?

Behaviour/demeanour/body language

- Matter of fact
- Not expecting skin and joint problem to be connected.

Issues for preparation of the case

If possible, nails should be painted.

Photos to show the doctor.

1 Picture of fungal/psoriasis fingernails with some typical pitting and onycholysis: http://www.dermnetnz.org/scaly/nail-psoriasis.html
2 Picture of scaly patchy rash elbows: http://www.dermnetnz.org/scaly/plaque-psoriasis.html

Materials for the doctor [displayed on the iPad in the CSA]

Case notes for the patient:

Name: Amelia Kowalski
Age: 35
Address: 2 Gull House

Social and family history

- Lives with partner
- Two children
- Non-smoker – drinks occasional vodka [1 shot socially only]

Past medical history

- Classical migraine 2001

Current medication

- Mirena coil
- Propranolol 40 mg – migraine prophylaxis

Other clinical details

Practice nurse 3 months ago.

- Well woman check all well – smear normal, coil threads seen.
- Propranolol working well for migraine.
- Rash back of elbow comes and goes, worried about her feet – suggest see doctor if no better.

CSA Case Marking Sheet: Case name: Amelia Kowalski [Case 10]	
Focus for the case: nail and skin as a possible presentation of systemic illness (psoriatic arthritis) in 35-year-old woman	
Data-gathering, technical and assessment skills	Take an organised history of nail and skin symptoms including other relevant medical social history Recognise skin and nail findings
Positive descriptors: • Takes a full history revealing social context of wet feet and bar work • Shows awareness of important co-morbidity, e.g. diabetes • Explores possibility of co-existing skin/nail problems, e.g. psoriasis/eczema asks about joint pains • Asks about PMH and drug history • Offers to examine feet and skin of elbows • Offer to take a nail scraping	**Negative descriptors:** • Disorganised unsystematic approach to history taking • Omits drug history • Does not gather relevant social or family history • Does not recognise the conditions from photographic evidence • Does not suggest or offer nail scraping
Clinical Management skills	Make correct diagnosis of nail and skin condition, i.e. fungal and co-existing psoriasis, negotiate appropriate investigation and offer treatments, referral and review

Positive descriptors: • Seeks to confirm the diagnosis by obtaining fungal scrapings • Makes a working diagnosis of fungal nail disease • Recognises the possibility of co-existing psoriatic nail disease and arthropathy • Explains the reasons why it is best to wait for test results, i.e. alternative or co-existing diagnosis and treatment choice • Explains about possible treatments and side effects – also beta-blocker link with psoriasis • Suggest blood test in relation to joint pains offers referral to dermatology/rheumatology • Recommends self-help leaflets • Arranges review	**Negative descriptors:** • Does not make diagnosis of fungal nail disease and/or recognise possibility of co-existing psoriasis presentation • Indiscriminately recommends oral drug treatment for fungal nail without considering further investigation or referral • Does not recognise possible worsening of rash symptoms as a drug side effect • Does not offer appropriate treatment for co-existing rash • Does not safety-net or offer review
Interpersonal skills	Demonstrate a professional and understanding approach to a problem-causing distress in the context of a person's working and family life
Positive descriptors: • Acknowledges the distress being caused by the symptoms • Empathic in impact of other possible diagnoses • Able to contain and manage uncertainty and work in partnership with patient • Recognises dilemma posed by beta-blockers which have helped migraine but may be making rash worse – evolves a plan around this	**Negative descriptors:** • Unsympathetic or dismissive of symptoms offers a wait and see approach • Lacks empathy in exploring alternative diagnoses • Does not work in partnership with patient to evolve a management plan

Name of the 'Patient'	Amelia Kowalski [Case 10]
Curriculum Clinical Statement	3.21 Care of people with skin conditions

This case is testing the candidate's ability to

- Make a correct working diagnosis and display awareness of differentials
- Negotiate a suitable management plan
- Show resourcefulness and take an opportunistic approach with a common problem
- Build relationship and trust with the patient.

Learning resources

http://www.rcgp.org.uk/gp-training-and-exams/~/media/Files/GP-training-and-exams/Curriculum-2012/RCGP-Curriculum-3-21-Skin-Problems.ashx.

http://cks.nice.org.uk/fungal-nail-infection#!topicsummary.

http://www.patient.co.uk/health/fungal-nail-infections-leaflet.

http://www.bad.org.uk/librarymedia/documents/Fungal%20infections%20of%20the%20nails%20Update%20Mar%202014%20-%20lay%20reviewed%20Mar%202014%20(corrected%20May%202014).pdf.

Case 11

Name of 'Patient': **Thomas Smith**
Gender: Male
Age: 61

Background

- Lives with his wife
- Two children aged 27 and 29 (both left home)
  Has worked 15 years for a medium-sized printing firm
- No undue stress but works long hours
- Wife works part-time in a school.

Opening statement

'My wife has booked this appointment for me because she's worried'
(You are nervous)

Information to give

Three days ago you had an episode lasting 15 minutes where you had weakness in your right arm and pins and needles on the right side of your face. This has resolved completely, and you have come for a check-up because your wife is worried.

Information to give, if asked specifically by the candidate

- Your speech was slightly slurred.
- Your eye did not close completely – only partial weakness in the eye lid.

The CSA Exam: Maximizing your Success, First Edition. Rachel Roberts.

Companion Website: www.wiley.com\go\Roberts\CSAExam

- These symptoms happened after lunch, and you had eaten a little more than usual and were sitting at your desk. Suddenly your right arm couldn't work the computer keyboard, and your face on the right side felt odd and different with pins and needles.
- No chest pain, no palpitations, no headache. No similar episodes in past.
- Did not affect swallowing.
- It did not affect your sense of smell or hearing.
- You were not confused.
- You did not lose your vision.
- You did not lose consciousness.
- You were not dizzy.
- You stopped smoking 1 year ago as you turned 60.
- You only drink alcohol socially.
  No regular medication.
- Your father had a stroke aged 64.
- You have driven to the surgery and parked the car on a meter outside the surgery.
- Patients ideas, concerns and expectations:

  I – you thought you had had a *probable mini stroke.*(checked on Google)
  C – you think you need blood tests and are *worried about having a stroke.*
  E – you want cholesterol and blood pressure checked and you *want a scan.*

Past medical history

- Age 18 – fractured wrist
- Age 34 – stress at work
- Age 55 – diverticulosis
- Medication – ispaghula husk 1 daily.

Expect the candidate to ask to examine you

Questions for the role-player to ask the doctor, if appropriate

- When you are told you should not drive – you are surprised and disappointed and ask the doctor why you can't drive although you fully recovered?
- Initially, you say you live around the corner and will drive home, if that's OK?
- If the doctor suggests you should not drive, do not resist and agree for your wife to pick you up.
- Question to ask, only if time permits – why did I have the mini-stroke?

Behaviour/demeanour/body language

- Concerned, co-operative and rather worried when TIA confirmed
- Disappointed when told you cannot drive.

Issues for preparation of the case

- Instructions to the person playing the 'Examiner':

  If the candidate offers to examine the patient, after the examination has been completed, please offer the appropriate card, or give the findings verbally appropriate to the examination undertaken.

  If only two people are doing the role-play, the 'Patient' will give the appropriate card or give the findings verbally appropriate to the examination undertaken.

Examination Card 1

- Pulse 74 regular
- BP 142/82
- Normal neurological examination

Examination Card 2

- No carotid bruits
- Heart sounds normal

Materials for the doctor [displayed on the iPad in the CSA]

Case notes for the patient:

Name:	Thomas Smith
Age:	61
Address:	24 Tilbury Road

Social and family history

- Lives with his wife

Past medical history

- Age 18 – fractured wrist
- Age 34 – stress at work
- Age 55 – diverticulosis

Current medication

- Medication – ispaghula husk 1 daily

CSA Case Marking Sheet: Case name: Thomas Smith [Case 11]	
Focus for the case: The candidate's ability to manage patient presenting with TIA, who is a driver. Arranging suitable treatment and management	
Data-gathering, technical and assessment skills	Gathers focused history and examination to confirm TIA diagnosis
Positive descriptors: • History gathers information to confirm TIA and exclude CVA • Focused history considers risk factors and social impact, especially driving • Explores impact on work and home • Examination is focused on cardiovascular risk • Good candidate picks up that he has driven to the surgery	**Negative descriptors:** • Disorganised gathering of data which does not appear guided by probabilities of disease • Focuses narrowly on the problem, e.g. only concentrating on TIA with no exploration of any other potential symptoms or causes • Examination does not include the relevant focused elements or is conducted with poor technique • Fails to discover he is a driver
Clinical Management skills	Shows awareness of correct management plan of TIA in a driver
Positive descriptors: • Explains diagnoses TIA rather than CVA • Arranges appropriate blood tests FBC, U+E, LFTs, TFT, Gluc, Lipids • Offers medication – aspirin and statin • Arranges referrals to TIA clinic • Follow-up after blood tests	**Negative descriptors:** • Candidate does not appear to reach appropriate differential diagnoses • Management not included appropriate blood tests • Failure to prescribe aspirin/statin • Failure to refer to TIA clinic • No follow-up arrangements

Interpersonal skills	Facilitates patients contribution and explains medical management, especially driving issue
Positive descriptors: • Active listening, and appropriately responds to his concerns and expectations of a scan • Provides relevant explanation of possible link of smoking and TIA • Maintains warmth, sympathy and understanding, while exploring the symptoms • Sensitively explains driving DVLA regulations	**Negative descriptors:** • Poor active listening skills • Causes unnecessary anxiety in the patient • Explanations of potential causes are not relevant or appropriate to the patient • Manner lacks warmth and understanding

Name of 'Patient'	Thomas Smith [Case 11]
Curriculum Clinical Statement	3.18 Care of People with Neurological Problems

This case is testing the candidate's ability to

- Confirm history of TIA and discover he is a driver
- Carry out relevant examination
- Assess cardiovascular risk
- Develop a safe management plan
- Prescribe appropriate medication
- Communicate sensitively the diagnosis and cessation of driving.

Learning resources

http://www.patient.co.uk/doctor/transient-ischaemic-attacks.
http://bestpractice.bmj.com/best-practice/monograph/107.htm.

Case 12

Name of 'Patient': **Debbie Wells**
Gender: Female
Age: 40

Background

- Single parent. Lives with her son aged 10.
- Works as secretary for international investment bank in the city.
- Divorced 5 years ago.

Opening statement

'My sleep is poor. I have been trying Nytol for the last few weeks and it is not working. Please could I have some sleeping tablets?'

Information to give

This year there has been performance management in the bank, and they are threatening to hold back a bonus because it is felt you have been late arriving to work on too many occasions and your performance has been below average.

Information to give, if asked specifically by the doctor

- Last few months have been very busy at work.
- You are worried about your 10-year-old son, who has important exams to gain entrance into selective secondary schools when aged 11.
- You go to sleep okay, but end up waking in the middle of the night and early morning and you are constantly thinking about work and your son.

The CSA Exam: Maximizing your Success, First Edition. Rachel Roberts.

Companion Website: www.wiley.com\go\Roberts\CSAExam

- You do not wake up refreshed in the mornings and find it difficult to concentrate at work.
- You have been under stress like this before when you were going through the divorce. However, this is different because you are having difficulty sleeping.
- You are often tearful after your son goes to sleep.
- Your mood is very low most of the time (on a scale from 1 to 10 – one being the lowest – your mood is between 3 and 4).
- At times, you wish you would not wake up but you have no active suicidal ideas.
- There is no past history of self-harm or suicidal ideas, and you have no intention of harming anyone.
- There has been no change in your appetite or weight, but you have lost interest in cooking which you used to enjoy.
- You have no hobbies because you're busy with work and your son.
- Being a single parent, you feel a major responsibility for your son.
- Your mother died 10 years ago but your elderly father lives locally and is fit for his age.
- You have one sister who lives in Scotland and is very supportive over the phone.
- You never smoked and only drink on special occasions.
- You are not self-medicating except for Nytol over the counter.
- Your ex-husband does not contact you and only makes contact with his son at Christmas.
- Patient's ideas, concerns and expectations:

  I – you thought, if sleep could be improved, you will get better.
  C – you think if your poor sleep carries on, your son will suffer and there's nothing you can do.
  E – you want sleeping tablets.

Past medical history

- Age 20 – Hay fever
- Age 35 – Divorced.

Medication

- Loratidine 10 mg mane (only during hay fever season)

Questions to ask the doctor, if appropriate

If offered antidepressants –

- Are they addictive? How soon will they work? Will they help my sleep?

If offered self-help therapy on the Internet or self-help books?

- You will accept these willingly.

If asked whether your employer can offer counselling –

- You did not consider this and will look into it.

If offered sleeping tablets –

- Can I take them daily?

If you are only offered lifestyle advice, then try to insist you would like medication for sleep because this will help you improve your concentration at work.

Behaviour/demeanour/body language

Good eye contact, normal speech, mood is low (and nearly tearful when talking about your son) No thought or perception disorder. Normal cognition and insight.

Concerned, co-operative and tired. Near to tears when discussing the possible school allocation for your son.

Body language, shoulders hunched and looking depressed.

Materials for the doctor [displayed on the iPad in the CSA]

Case notes for the patient:

Name:	Debbie Wells
Age:	40
Address:	62 Moat Lane

Social and family history

- Lives with son

Past medical history

Age 20 – Hay fever

Age 35 – Divorced.

Medication

Loratidine 10 mg mane (only during hay fever season)

CSA Case Marking Sheet: Case name: Debbie Wells [Case 12]	
Focus for the case: The candidate's ability to manage a patient presenting with depression, who is a single parent. Arranging suitable treatment and management for both.	
Data-gathering, technical and assessment skills	Demonstrates a structured approach to diagnosis of depression and excludes suicidal ideas
Positive descriptors: • Gathers information to confirm depression and excludes suicidal ideation • Focused history considering risk factors and impact of son's future • Explores impact on work and home • Mental state examination focused and shows good insight	**Negative descriptors:** • Disorganised gathering of data which does not appear guided by probabilities of disease • Focuses narrowly on the problem – does not consider importance of son's school • Mental state examination done poorly • Fails to ascertain suicidal ideation
Clinical Management skills	Demonstrates appropriate management of depression
Positive descriptors: • Explains diagnoses of depression and stress related to son's school placement. • Offers self-help and counselling or IAPT. • Offers medication –antidepressant, e.g. mirtazapine • Safety-nets, if suicidal • Arranges follow-up in 3 to 4 weeks • Offers voluntary organisations, e.g. CAB for financial advice and MIND	**Negative descriptors:** • Candidate does not appear to reach the diagnosis of depression or stress • Management does not include self-help, counselling • Failure to prescribe antidepressant • Failure to offer voluntary organisations • Follow-up arrangements not specified

Interpersonal skills	Sensitively explores issues with her son. Recognises psychological and social impact of diagnosis.
Positive descriptors: • Active listening, and appropriately responds to her concerns and reassures • Provides relevant explanation of depression and links to work and her son • Maintains warmth, sympathy and understanding, while exploring the symptoms • Sensitively explores suicidal ideation • With empathy explains protective factors of her family • A good candidate may explain self-help and lifestyle advice	**Negative descriptors:** • Poor active listening skills • Causes unnecessary anxiety in the patient and poor explanation of depression • Fails to explore how the patient's life is affected by her symptoms • Manner lacks warmth and understanding • Insensitive discussion of suicidal ideation • Fails to recognise impact of her son's future school

Name of 'Patient': **Debbie Wells** [Case 12]
Curriculum Clinical Statement: 3.10 Care of People with Mental Health Problems

This case is testing the candidate's ability to

- Confirm history of depression and exclude suicidal ideation
- Carry out mental state examination
- Develop a safe management plan and prescribe appropriate medication
- Communicate sensitively the diagnosis
- Encourage mother to consider self-help.

Learning resources

http://www.patient.co.uk/doctor/depression-pro.

http://www.rcpsych.ac.uk/mentalhealthinfoforall/problems/depression/depression.aspx.

https://www.nice.org.uk/search?q=Depression.

http://bestpractice.bmj.com/best-practice/monograph/55.html.

Case 13

Name of 'Patient': Ashia Pollock
Gender: Female
Age: 11

Background

- Lives with parents
- Mother originally from Ethiopia – works as senior nurse in ITU
- Father originally from Devon – works as manager in IT firm
- Ashia is in her final year at local junior school
  Mother is attending alone because Ashia is at school.

Opening statement

'Hello doctor, I just need a referral to the skin specialist for Ashia'

Information to give

Ashia has been seen twice in the last 2 months, and the last doctor did suggest she would benefit from referral to a skin specialist if the steroid cream did not work.

Information to give, if asked specifically by the doctor

- Ashia has had eczema since she was 3 or 4 years old, but it has always been mild and easily controlled with moisturiser.
- In the past, there have been no trigger factors.

The CSA Exam: Maximizing your Success, First Edition. Rachel Roberts.

Companion Website: www.wiley.com\go\Roberts\CSAExam

- Ashia applies E45 herself once or twice a day, and mother applies steroid twice a day.
- Ashia's eczema was relatively well controlled until 2 months ago using the moisturiser once a day.
- Now, particularly on her arms and legs and patches on her trunk, her skin is getting dry and itchy.
- She sometimes wakes up in the night, and mother has to apply either the moisturising cream or the steroid.
- When she saw the first doctor about 2 months ago, she was advised to use the steroid called hydrocortisone 1% twice a day and the moisturiser.
- When she saw the second doctor about a month ago, she was given a stronger steroid – eumovate – to use twice a day and the moisturiser.
- There has been no change in the soap, shampoo or washing powder in the last 2 months.
- *If asked directly* – how often do you apply the e45 moisturiser? – reply once a day, especially when using the steroids.
- If Dr asks for mother to bring Ashia in, say that her skin is exactly the same as the previous two occasions when seen by doctors in the same surgery.
- If the Dr suggests checking for infection because you're a nurse, you are aware there is no obvious skin infection.
- *If asked directly* about changes in last 2 months – you will admit to giving Ashia a healthier diet. You introduced wholemeal bread and more nuts
- Mother's ideas, concerns and expectations –

  I – You think it may be allergy.

  C – You are concerned because steroid is lightening skin in patches – not cosmetically acceptable on Ashia's dark skin. Itching at night is not good because next few months are important at school as she has entrance exams for selective secondary schools.

  E – You want a referral to a specialist.

Questions to ask the doctor, if appropriate

- Will the patches on Ashia's skin, which have lost some colour due to the steroids, recover?
- Will you refer to the paediatrician or the dermatologist?
- Do you think she will need allergy testing?

Past medical history

- Age 18 months – admitted viral-induced wheeze

Ashia's medication

- E45 cream qds prn
- Hydrocortisone 1% (acute prescription)
- Eumovate (clobetasone butyrate) (acute prescription)

Family history

- Ashia's father has history of asthma and hay fever.

Behaviour/demeanour/body language

Concerned, co-operative and willing to accept the doctor's management as long as it includes referral.

Will ask for allergy testing but not insist.

Will be surprised when told wholemeal bread and nuts can cause allergy and eczema.

Materials for the doctor [displayed on the iPad in the CSA]

Case notes for the patient

Name:	Ashia Pollock
Age:	11
Address:	56 Stock Lane

Social and family history

- Lives with parents
- Mother originally from Ethiopia – works as senior nurse in ITU
- Father originally from Devon – works as manager in IT firm
- Ashia in her final year at local junior school.

Past medical history

- Age 18 months – admitted viral-induced wheeze

Current medication

- E45 cream qds prn
- Hydrocortisone 1% (acute prescription)
- Eumovate (clobetasone butyrate) (acute prescription)

Previous consultations

- 2 months ago
  Generalised eczema especially limbs and trunk – not infected – add hydrocortisone.
- 1 month ago
  Eczema same – not improving – add Eumovate and possibly refer

CSA Case Marking Sheet: Case name: Ashia Pollock [Case 13]	
Focus for the case: The candidate's ability to manage parent presenting with a child with recent exacerbation of eczema. Arranging suitable treatment and management	
Data-gathering, technical and assessment skills	Gathers focused history and examination to confirm dietary exacerbation and compliance with moisturiser exacerbating eczema
Positive descriptors: • Gathers information to confirm how often creams are applied • Focused history considers risk factors for atopy and recent dietary changes • Explores impact on sleep and school • Examination is offered as patient not present – to exclude infection • Good candidate picks up frequency of moisturiser application and diet change	**Negative descriptors:** • Disorganised gathering of data, fails to identify application frequency of moisturiser • Focuses narrowly on the problem and not identify dietary change • Examination not offered • Fails to discover family history of atopy
Clinical Management skills	Shows awareness of correct management of eczema and dietary exacerbation due to food intolerance

Positive descriptors: • Explains diagnoses most probable reaction to dietary change • Arranges for mother to keep food and drink diary • Explains qds application of moisturiser • Offers night-time antihistamine • Depending on confidence of Dr in managing eczema may or may not arrange referral to paediatric clinic • Explains allergy testing may be done by paediatric clinic after the food and drink diary information • Follow-up after 3 to 4 wks with child	**Negative descriptors:** • Candidate does not appear to reach appropriate diagnoses • Management includes stronger steroid • Fails to explain qds application of E45 • Failure to prescribe antihistamine. • Fails to explain adequately reason for non-referral to paediatric clinic • Fails to explain context of allergy testing. • No follow-up arrangements
Interpersonal skills	Facilitates parent's contribution and explains medical management, taking account of mothers concerns
Positive descriptors: • Active listening, and appropriately responds to concerns about steroids causing lighter skin patches • Provides relevant explanation of possible link of dietary change and eczema • Maintains warmth, sympathy and understanding, while exploring the symptoms • Take into consideration the impact on sleep and school performance	**Negative descriptors:** • Poor active listening skills. • Causes unnecessary anxiety in the parent by prescribing stronger steroid • Explanations of potential causes such as dietary and frequency of moisturiser not explained with sensitivity • Manner lacks warmth and understanding of the impact on school and sleep

Name of the 'Patient':	**Ashia Pollock** [Case 13]
Curriculum Clinical Statements:	3.04 Care of children and young people 3.21 Care of people with skin problems

This case is testing the candidate's ability to

- Confirm history of eczema and dietary exacerbation
- Offer examination at next appointment
- Develop a safe management plan and prescribe appropriate medication
- Communicate sensitively that the exacerbation may be dietary related
- Address parental concerns.

Learning resources

http://www.patient.co.uk/doctor/atopic-dermatitis-and-eczema.

http://pathways.nice.org.uk/pathways/atopic-eczema-in-children.

'Management of difficult and severe eczema in childhood' BMJ 2012; 345.e4770 (Published 23 July 2012).

Case 14

Name of patient: **Olu Wa-Simba**
Afro Caribbean: child is a male, consults with parent – mother
Ages: child aged 8–11 years – mother aged 25–35

Background

Mother is a single parent, but they live with grandparents who look after Olu, as mother works in a local bank in the mortgage department. She is able to drop him to school but grandparents pick up after-school.

Olu has a sister named Elizabeth – who is 2 years younger. He gets on OK with her and is protective of his younger sister.

Olu attends Croft Green Primary School.

He likes school and wants to be a policeman (such as his grand dad was) when he grows up.

Despite his asthma, he does well at football and plays for the school football team.

Opening statement (given by mother)

'I have been asked to make an appointment so that I can have a repeat of his blue inhaler'

If asked – 'Tell me more'

'He uses his blue inhaler everyday and that sorts out his cough'

The CSA Exam: Maximizing your Success, First Edition. Rachel Roberts.

Companion Website: www.wiley.com\go\Roberts\CSAExam

Past medical history

Asthma since aged 2
Eczema – resolved by age 4.

Information to give freely if asked

Asthma –

- He uses his blue inhaler two or three times everyday.
- You can't remember when he last had a check-up, but it was sometime last year.
- He has a cough daily and that's why he uses his blue inhaler.
- He suffers from a cough at night a couple times a week and occasionally uses the blue inhaler.
- At school, the teachers let him take the blue inhaler that helps.
- He only gets wheeze when he has a bad cold or chest infection.
- He does not suffer from shortness of breath.

His medication for asthma

- He is taking the brown inhaler one puff ABOUT twice a day. (Mother looks sheepish – because she knows he sometimes misses it in the morning as it's a hurry to get him to school.)

If asked what you mean ABOUT twice a day –

- You will admit freely in the mornings, it is difficult to get two kids ready and get them to school on time and, therefore, occasionally – two, three times a week – the brown inhaler is missed in the morning. But you always make sure he has it in the evening.
- He always uses the inhalers directly into his mouth.

If asked why he does not use the aero chamber –

- It takes longer to use the chamber and he feels embarrassed using the aero chamber at school in front of the other kids.

If specifically asked

Family history – mother and grandmother have asthma.
Mother smokes at home, usually tries to smoke outdoors.

Expect the candidate to ask to examine Olu

If Dr asks to do his peak flow – you will let him, and we expect the doctor to explain to Olu how to use the peak flow meter.

(Before Olu actually uses the peak flow meter – the examiner will say this is 'normal'.)

The Dr may ask if Olu has his inhaler. Mother will say he has left it at home as you live around the corner and he has run out of his last blue inhaler.

If the Dr asks to get Olu's height and weight – the examiner will tell the Dr – 'Height 70th centile and weight 50th centile'.

If the Dr asks to check how Olu uses inhaler –

Mother can say this was checked last time and he was advised to use the aero chamber.

Dr may ask you to demonstrate how Olu uses his inhaler with an aero chamber.

Need to instruct mother how to demonstrate this

Questions for the role-player to ask the doctor if appropriate

'Can he have tablets for his asthma rather than inhalers?'

If the Dr asks what tablets. You can say your friend's child has asthma and hay fever and they were given tablets starting with the letter M – you think they're called Monty? These tablets have been very helpful.

Behaviour/demeanour/body language

Olu brings in a comic and spends sometime looking at the pictures while Dr is obtaining history from his mother. Forthcoming if asked questions directly, but otherwise lets his mother do the talking. Co-operative if the doctor asks to do the peak flow.

Mother – Calm, co-operative and feels guilty that she still smokes, but was not aware that smoking indoors would make his asthma worse.

Issues for preparation of the case

- Instructions to the person playing the 'Examiner':

If the Dr asks to examine Olu's chest – say this is 'normal'.

Olu's peak flow – expect the doctor to explain to Olu how to use the peak flow meter, but before Olu actually uses the peak flow meter – say this is 'normal'.

If the Dr asks to get Olu's height and weight – tell the Dr – 'Height 70th centile and weight 50th centile'.

Materials for the doctor [displayed on the iPad in the CSA]

Case notes for the patient:

Name:	Olu Wa-Simba
Age:	8
Address:	41 Euston Drive

Social background

Single parent
1 sibling, sister 2 years younger

Past medical history

Age 2 – asthma
Age 18 months – eczema – resolved by age 4.

Current medication

Beclomethasone inhaler 50 mcg 1 or 2 puffs bd
Salbutamol inhaler 200 mcg 1 or 2 puffs qds
Aero chamber x1

Previous consultations

3 years ago – Asthma suboptimal control – advice given.
18 months ago – Asthma affects sports and nocturnal cough. Advice on use of medication and aero chamber.

CSA Case Marking Sheet: Case name: Olu Wa-Simba [Case 14]	
Focus for the case: Recognise need for asthma review in context of child's school and home circumstances.	
Data-gathering, technical and assessment skills	Demonstrates structured history and examination relevant to asthma review, with particular attention to social history
Positive descriptors: • History elucidates asthma poorly controlled • Focused history – details, asthma symptoms review • Asks how aero chamber is used • Explores possible differential diagnoses – e.g. mother's smoking and compliance with inhalers • Examination is focused on peak flow, height and weight • Good candidate asks if anyone smokes at home and checks social history	**Negative descriptors:** • Disorganised gathering of data which does not appear guided by probabilities of disease • Focuses narrowly on the problem, e.g. only concentrating on inhaler technique or compliance with no exploration of any other potential symptoms or causes • Does not ask about cough, wheeze and shortness of breath for asthma • Does not consider social history • Examination does not include peak flow, height, weight and inhaler technique and via aero chamber
Clinical Management skills	Demonstrates the involvement of child and mother in compliance with medication and improved understanding of asthma

Positive descriptors: • Recognises no asthma review in the last 12 months; checks inhaler technique; offers advice on step up and step down for steroid inhaler • Explains aero chamber technique • Prescribes an extra one for school • Offers follow-up either with the asthma nurse or doctor in 1 or 2 months	• Candidate does not appear to reach appropriate diagnoses • Fails to manage asthma • Issues prescription for Ventolin with no review or limited review • Does not explain regular use of beclomethasone • Does not show use of aero chamber • Does not offer open appointment for follow-up if asthma symptoms get worse
Interpersonal skills	Having recognised poor asthma control, sensitively explains inhaler technique and educates mother regarding smoking and medication compliance
Positive descriptors: • Active listening, and responds appropriately to requests • Interacts at appropriate level with child • Provides relevant explanation re. treatment & the duration and reassures mother • Maintains warmth and understanding while exploring the symptoms and possible causes	**Negative descriptors:** • Poor active listening skills. • Causes unnecessary anxiety in the patient or parent • Poor interaction with child • Explanations of potential causes are not relevant or appropriate to the patient • Manner lacks warmth and understanding

Name of the 'Patient': **Olu Wa-Simba** [Case 14]
Curriculum Clinical Statement: 3 04 Care of children and young people
3 19 Respiratory Health
3 01 Healthy people, promoting health and preventing disease

This case is testing the candidate's ability to

- Recognise poor asthma control
- Carry out an asthma review
- Be aware of the social background of mother and child
- Interact appropriately with both parent and child.

Learning resources

British Thoracic Society, 17 Doughty Street, London WC1N 2PL, www.brit-thoracic.org.uk.

Scottish Intercollegiate Guidelines Network, Gyle Square, 1 South Gyle Crescent, Edinburgh EH12 9EB.

British guideline on the management of asthma. Quick Reference Guide. First published 2003. Revised edition published 2014. SIGN and the BTS consent to the photocopying of this QRG for the purpose of implementation in the NHS in England, Wales, Northern Ireland and Scotland.

Case 15

Name of 'Patient': **Nilesh Patel**
Gender: Male
Age: 11 years 4 months
Ethnicity: Asian
Attends with Dad: Mr Sunil Patel [37]

Background

- Lives with Mum and Dad and younger sister Alicia.
- Attends school nearby Beech Park.
- Wants to do sports apprenticeship after GCSEs, has ambitions to be a professional cricketer.
- Dad runs chain of successful grocery stores and is a property developer.
- He is cricket mad.
- Mum (also British Asian) helps in the business and runs one of the shops, but is also training to become a nurse.

Opening statement

> [Father] *'It's his legs, Doctor, he's been getting odd pains in them for the last few months'*

As they enter, Nilesh is playing with his phone. After greeting the doctor, Dad does the talking initially, but in response to questions from the doctor, Dad asks Nilesh to put his phone away and speak to the doctor. Nilesh compliantly stops and engages in responses.

The CSA Exam: Maximizing your Success, First Edition. Rachel Roberts.

Companion Website: www.wiley.com\go\Roberts\CSAExam

Information to give

- Legs have been aching in the thighs and shins now and again for the last few months.
- Worse in the evening after sports sometimes.
- Most recently a dull ache in the thighs after cricket nets lasted a few hours last weekend and was waking him up – better after nurofen.
- Had same last year at the end of the cricket season – then settled down on its own.
- Rest helps.

Information to give, if asked specifically by the candidate

- No fever, otherwise well now
- No limp, 'they just ache'
- No recent preceding or associated viral/flu-like illness
- No family history of joint problems, no family history of TB
- No pain in testicles, no waterworks symptoms (no pain when you wee, or blood in wee, or going more often)
- No back pain. No pain or tenderness in knee
- Appetite and weight ok – not vegetarian
- Developmental checks all ok – height and growth normal
- You have never had any blood tests – don't like sound of it, but would go for one, if doctor says it's a good idea.

Examination

Expect to be examined. The doctor should examine your knee and your hip, so expect this – have football shorts on under tracksuit/or be wearing shorts.

All joints have a full range of movement – there is no local tenderness – basically it all seems normal now.

Questions for the role-players to ask the doctor, if appropriate

- *Does he need any further tests at the moment? – a scan or something?*
- *(If vitamin D hasn't been mentioned) – Mum was diagnosed with vitamin D deficiency on a blood test recently and she was a bit worried about Nilesh's legs. …*
- Could it be anything to do with the blood? … if doctor probes … your wife has been googling about it and came up with 'blood things'.

Behaviour/demeanour/body language

[Nilesh]

Asian athletic build. NOT overweight (high BMI would increase suspicion of SUFE).

Cheerful, a bit vague, sporty tracksuit, fiddling with phone which you switch off when dad tells you to as you walk in. Look to dad to answer when you don't. You prefer cricket to football.

You like school and have no problems there. There is no bullying.

You don't want to stop playing cricket, but would be prepared to reduce your activity a bit if the doctor advises it.

You have no idea about your parents' worry about leukaemia. If this gets broached, for example conversation about blood – become concerned – a boy at school had a blood problem last year … and is having treatment for leukaemia.

[Dad]

Business man type, casual shirt but no tie. Second-generation British Asian. Respectful to doctor but not overdeferential. Proud of son and worried re. symptoms. Wife (training to be a nurse) has googled symptoms and is worried about leukaemia. Dad thinks this is absurd – but is slightly worried about it.

Issues for preparation of the case

- Instructions to the person playing the 'Examiner':

The candidate should conduct a proficient examination of the knee and hip excluding local tenderness and confirming full range of movement, internal and external rotation of hip, check gait.

After examination has been completed, please offer the card, or give verbally the findings appropriate to the examination undertaken.

Examination Card

Apyrexial
BCG scar present
If candidate asks, rest of examination normal.

Materials for the doctor [displayed on the iPad in the CSA]

Case notes for the patient

Name:	Nilesh Patel
Age:	11 years
Address:	14 Cover Drive

Social and family history

- Lives with Mum and Dad and younger sister
- Attends Beech Park School.

Past medical history

- None

Current medication

- Nil

Other clinical details

- No allergies
- Fully immunised
- BCG – as infant

CSA Case Marking Sheet: Case name: Nilesh Patel [Case 15]	
Focus for the case: The importance of the presentation is that there are a number of serious things it could be, but is likely growing pains/ recurrent nocturnal limb pain and possible vitamin D deficiency	
Data-gathering, technical and assessment skills	Demonstrate ability to take an adequate general and orthopaedic history from an 11-year boy and father
Positive descriptors: • Establishes the reason for attendance • Asks about fever, limp timing, general health • Takes social history/school/ home • Family history • Covers immunisation • Touches on TB/BCG and vitamin D deficiency as possibilities • Conducts adequate exam – hip knee 'joint above and below' • Suggests possible further tests if symptoms persist	**Negative descriptors:** • Fails to explore more widely, narrow in range of questions • Makes assumptions about diagnosis • Does not ask about medical risk factors • Does not examine hip and knee adequately
Clinical Management skills	Offers appropriate and comprehensive advice and review

Positive descriptors: • Adequately establishes no active symptoms and signs today • Recommends follow-up with self and/or other team members • Suggests a symptom diary and review • Recommends blood test but compliant with child declining it for now • Suggests XR not helpful at present • Touches on growing pains/recurrent nocturnal limb pain as possibility	**Negative descriptors:** • Prescribes inappropriately • Fails to assess risk • Fails to give opportunistic advice • Gives wrong advice • Fails to safety-net • Fails to offer follow-up • Recommends XR
Interpersonal skills	Puts young person at ease and involves them in management decisions; maintains effective working relationship
Positive descriptors: • Establishes rapport and maintains professional approach • Covers any issue of confidentiality and puts patient at ease • Promotes involvement and inclusion of parent and child in decision making and choices • Elicits concerns re. leukaemia and reassures appropriately	**Negative descriptors:** • Fails to form rapport while maintaining a professional and comprehensive approach, e.g. negative in response to mobile phone • General approach likely to deter young person from seeking advice again • Insists on blood tests, X-rays, further tests which child not keen on

Name of the patient: **Nilesh Patel** [Case 15]
Curriculum Clinical Statement: 3.04 Care of Children and Young People

This case is testing the candidate's ability to

- Gain the trust of a young patient
- Take a history that covers likely red flag diagnoses
- Examine appropriately
- Communicate information
- Formulate a management plan that recognises possible diagnoses
- Demonstrate social and cultural sensitivity.

Learning needs/resources

Consider – slipped upper femoral epiphysis, perthes, growing pains vitamin D deficiency in vulnerable groups

Arthritis Research Campaign. (2008) Hands On – Growing pains: a practical guide for primary care. http://www.arthritisresearchuk.org/shop/products/publications/information-for-medical-professionals/hands-on/series-6-x-stock/ho1-series-6.aspx.

Vitamin D deficiency in children – An up-to-the-minute and user-friendly summary is available at https://www.rnoh.nhs.uk/clinical-services/paediatric-adolescents/vitamin-d-children.

Widen your thinking about and learning from this case:

Slipped upper femoral epiphysis – review article. Peck D. Slipped capital femoral epiphysis: diagnosis and management. Am Fam Physician. 2010; 82(3): 258–262.

Perthes Disease. GP notebook provides a good overview. http://www.gpnotebook.co.uk/simplepage.cfm?ID=1657798668.

Case 16

Name of 'Patient': **Stephanie Caldwell**
Gender: Female
Age: 10

Background

- Lives with both parents, Jean and Steven
- Has 1 older brother, Robert age 14
- Attends Grange Green primary school

Opening statement

> *'I've been having these really bad headaches, so my mum says I should come and see the Doctor'*
>
> Stephanie

> *'I've taken the morning off work to bring Stephanie, as nothing I've suggested seems to be working'*
>
> Jean (mother)

Information to give

- You have had headaches for around 4 weeks.
- Before that you were clear of them for 2–3 months, but again before this you had them for 4–5 weeks.
- They are happening everyday.
- They are at the front and back of your head.
- They have occasionally been bad enough to stop you going to school.
- A few times a week, you have to take paracetamol or nurofen.

The CSA Exam: Maximizing your Success, First Edition. Rachel Roberts.

Companion Website: www.wiley.com\go\Roberts\CSAExam

Information to give if asked about accompanying symptoms or things which affect the headaches

- You are not sick with the headaches.
- You do not have any changes in eyesight with them.
- They are there usually by lunch time.
- You have no other symptoms at all.
- Nothing seems to make them better or worse, except sometimes a tablet helps.
- They developed after the flu the first time, but just seemed to carry on.
- Mother can respond, if asked, that there is no FH of headaches.

Information to give, if asked specifically by the doctor

- Your parents both work long hours in the city.
- When needed, you have a child minder after school.
- Your brother is well and you get on well with him.
- You have just this week finished entrance exams for a selective secondary school, which your parents are very keen for you to pass.
- You had revision sessions with tutors which started a few months ago for preparation.
- You want to become a vet, and so are a little worried, as you want to succeed.
- You have not been sleeping quite as well recently.
- You have friends at school, and no bullying.
- You are a hard worker.
- You do not have specific hobbies, but will join in with usual school activities.

Questions to ask the doctor, if appropriate

- Can you give me some medicine to stop this?
- Mother – I really don't want Stephanie to be struggling through school in pain, what can you do?
- Mother – Does she need any tests to see why this is happening?
- Mother – Should she have a scan, Doctor?

Behaviour/demeanour/body language

Stephanie – You are quiet and co-operative, not really smiling, but calm. You will smile and show some relief if it is clear that the doctor is offering help to resolve the problem. You will seem worried or disappointed if the doctor does not seem to know why this is happening, or just says it is tension and does not seem to help you stop the problem. If the doctor asks to refer you to a specialist, you will look worried and ask why – but agree to it.

Mother, Jean – smiling at outset, calm and allows Stephanie to speak, but interjects if it seems no action is being taken. Jean is assertive in asking for tests, or a clear solution.

Issues for preparation of the case

- Instructions to the person playing the 'Examiner':

After examination has been completed, please offer the card, or give the findings appropriate to the examination undertaken.

If only two people are doing the role-play, the 'Patient' will give the card, or give the findings appropriate to the examination undertaken.

Examination Card

Fundoscopy normal, cranial nerves and neurology normal
Ears, nose and throat normal
No sign of anaemia, no other abnormalities.

Materials for the doctor [displayed on the iPad in the CSA]

Case notes for the patient:

Name:	Stephanie Caldwell
Age:	10
Address:	12 Fairview Road

Social and family history

Parents are patients of the practice, Jean aged 40, Steven aged 42. No significant past medical history

Brother, Robert, aged 14, no significant past medical history

Stephanie – Past Medical History: Nil

Case Marking Sheet: Case name: Stephanie Caldwell [Case 16]	
Focus for the case: Communicate effectively with a 10-year-old girl and her mother. Ascertain most likely cause is tension headache. Use good interpersonal skills to help guide Stephanie and her mother in the management of this problem	
Data-gathering, technical and assessment skills	Obtains appropriate history, social factors, and seeks appropriate examination
Positive descriptors: • Obtains clear history of the time course of the illness • Asks for any relevant associated features of the headache and excludes red flags • Obtains relevant social history and pressures experienced by Stephanie • Seeks appropriate examination data • Reaches conclusion likely diagnosis is tension headache. May seek to exclude migraine	**Negative descriptors:** • Disorganised history, no clear picture of timeline • Does not exclude red flags or check for relevant associated features of the headache • Does not obtain the history of exams and pressure • Does not offer appropriate examination • Does not make correct differential diagnosis
Clinical Management skills	Avoids excessive investigations; arranges appropriate management plan for tension headaches
Positive descriptors: • Discusses the link between tension and headaches • Discusses reasons why other diagnoses are less likely • May arrange a headache diary • May arrange basic checks to exclude other causes, such as optician's check • Does not refer to paediatrics nor for scanning in the first instance	**Negative descriptors:** • Does not explain the potential link between tension and headaches • Does not explore differential diagnosis with patient and family • Does not seek to corroborate potential diagnosis of tension headache • Refers to out-patient clinic or arranges scanning

Interpersonal skills	Ability to collaborate with mother and daughter over management of tension and presenting symptoms
Positive descriptors: • Engages effectively and with empathy with Stephanie • Engages effectively and with empathy with her mother Jean • Is able to ascertain from Stephanie the majority of the information • Is able to be reassuring about the causes of the headache • Seeks to develop shared agreement about the causes of tension and possible solutions • Stephanie and her mother are given room to ask questions and share their thoughts	**Negative descriptors:** • Communication with Stephanie lacking in empathy or ineffective • Communication with mother lacking in empathy, or ineffective • Is not able to ascertain most of the information directly from Stephanie • Does not manage to reassure effectively • Does not reach an agreed shared management plan regarding the causes of tension • Does not develop a shared management plan, or is doctor-centred

Name of the 'Patient': **Stephanie Caldwell** [Case 16]
Curriculum Clinical Statement: 3.04 Care of children and young people

This case is testing the candidate's ability to

- Communicate effectively with a parent and child
- Address difficulty arising from social issues with a parent and child
- Gather data well and reach an appropriate differential diagnosis in a child with headaches
- Make appropriate decisions around the need for investigation in a child with headaches
- Use good interpersonal skills with both mother and child to help manage tension headaches.

Learning resources

Headaches in young children and adults (NICE, Sept 2012, endorsed by Royal College of Paediatrics and Child health, Oct' 2013) CG 150. https://www.nice.org.uk/guidance/cg150.

In terms of considering or excluding more serious causes of headache in children: "The diagnosis of brain tumours in children" by The Brain Tumour Charity, endorsed by RCPCH, version 3, March 2011. http://connect.qualityincare.org/__data/assets/pdf_file/0004/553981/Quick_Ref_Guide.pdf.

"Headache: tension type" by Clinical Knowledge Summaries/NICE. http://cks.nice.org.uk/headache-tension-type.

Index

The CSA Exam: Maximizing your Success, First Edition. Rachel Roberts.

Companion Website: www.wiley.com\go\Roberts\CSAExam